This book is dedicated to my children;

Joseph, Kevin, Sean and Patrick....I Love You.

and

to my wife, Lisamarie,

without whom this book and my life would not be complete.

I love you.

JH

ACKNOWLEDGMENTS

I would like to thank Dana Osler and Valerie Muehleman for their hard work and research.

I would also like to thank Gaston Perez, M.D. for his support and encouragement. James Johnston, M.D. and Frank Hart, M.D. for their knowledge, insight and friendship; Tom Little for his help and expertise. Richard Becker, M. D. for his many years of friendship and support. And Dr. John McGurty for being Dr. John McGurty.

I would also like to thank Cheryl and Vinnie Malaspina, Jeff Rundle, Lenny Catalino and Gus Mohammed for their friendship, weight loss and encouragement. And to my patients who have encouraged me by their weight loss and improved health.

And most especially, to Paul M. Long, M.D. my partner and friend, for his encouragement and prodding.

JH

First Printing December 1998

Photography by Melanie Blount

Printing by Perry Printing Co., Inc.

CONTENTS

Introduction

Obesity is the cause of most of our health problems. There is no argument among physicians that it contributes to 90% of the Hypertension, Diabetes of Adult Onset and Cardiovascular Disease that we deal with on a daily basis. The difference is *how* we approach this problem. Getting people to lose weight is crucial to their health. There are two basic philosophies to treat obesity.

The first camp and the vast majority prescribe a low fat, and calorie restricted diet. The theory is based on the calorie and the type of calorie. You need to take in fewer calories than you burn and you need to avoid high caloric foods such as saturated fats and cholesterol. This eliminates most meats, cheese and eggs. It relies upon complex carbohydrates such as pasta, whole grains, vegetables and fruits. This is supposed to make us healthier and slim. IT DOESN'T WORK!

I bought that philosophy for 15 years and I practiced it on my patients, they didn't get better. They got fatter, their sugars went higher, their cholesterols went higher, their blood pressures went higher. I tried to fix all of the broken parts with pills. A pill for your blood pressure, a pill for your cholesterol, and pills and/or insulin for your diabetes. They continued to gain more and more weight, and I continued to get more and more frustrated with them. The American Heart Association recommends it, The American Dietetic Association recommends it and The American Diabetes Association recommends it. The problem is - IT DOESN'T WORK.

After some key eye opening adventures I have had with my patients, my eyes are finally open. If it doesn't work, I am not going to use it. My patients have demonstrated to me that IT DOESN'T WORK. To put a diabetic on a low-fat high carbohydrate diet is ridiculous. Carbohydrates are sugar, SUGAR is what they have trouble handling. But it is very difficult for a conservative physician to break tradition. There are well-meaning researchers who feel it is very important not to eat fat. But they're WRONG. Carbohydrates are the enemy, carbohydrates make people fat. They induce hormonal changes in the blood that promote fat storage and restrict fat utilization for energy. Carbohydrates are such a good fuel that we don't have to rely on all of that fuel we have stored. Our fat is never called into play or utilized because we don't need it. What I finally realized was that you can induce your metabolism to work *for* you, rather than *against* you. That's what this philosophy is going to teach you. Avoid carbohydrates and you will lose weight very quickly and efficiently. In the process of losing weight you will improve your blood pressure, your cholesterol, your physical conditioning, and your outlook on life.

Three issued need to be addressed:

Does it work?

Is it safe?

How do I do it?

I will address these issues in the forthcoming chapters. I will try to make it easy to understand because a great deal of this has required very intricate research in very complicated matters such as cholesterol, insulin resistance and the like.

This is written for my patients as a handbook on how to proceed with easy weight loss and in the process a healthier lifestyle. But because my primary goal is the safety of my patients, I will explain why it is safe and healthy to eat more fat and to restrict carbohydrates.

The weight loss that we have achieved with this diet is unprecedented. I have also after several hundred patients, not seen a failure. The bottom line is you have to check your cholesterol's and your blood sugars before and after you've done this for three months. That is the proof in the pudding. If it helps you, than certainly the weight loss is an added benefit and it works. If it doesn't, than I am wrong.

Most of my patients prior to their low carbohydrate, insulin regulating diet were spinning their wheels, gaining weight with no improvement in their medical problems. That is all changed now and it is exciting to watch. There is hope for every obese person. You don't need to continue on with the same course.

I wish you the best of health and I know your weight loss will be very satisfying.

CHAPTER I.

CHOLESTEROL PHOBIA - THE WRONG ENEMY

A *phobia* is an irrational, excessive and persistent fear of some thing or situation. If you have a phobia of close spaces, you fear and avoid them (claustrophobia). If you are phobic in crowds, you are agoraphobic. America has become CHOLESTEROL PHOBIC. For the last twenty years, we have been avoiding fat and cholesterol with increasing eagerness. During this time we have been getting fatter and fatter. Obesity is now present in 33% of Americans. This is defined as the body mass index greater than 20% of your ideal weight. The body mass index is probably the best way to calculate obesity. Body mass index equals weight in kilograms divided by height in meters, squared.

We have been following a low fat, high complex carbohydrate diet for at least 20 years now. We have targeted cholesterol and saturated fat as the enemy. The level of obesity, however, during this time has climbed from 20% to 33% of our population in the United States. Your enemy is <u>not</u> fat. To my amazement, carbohydrates create higher cholesterol's than eating pure fat. The problem is BODY fat. Anything you eat that creates increased body fat, will make your cholesterol numbers worse and affect your heart, blood pressure, and kidneys accordingly. Whatever we can do to get rid of body fat, will help our cholesterol, blood pressure, blood sugar, and heart. If you eat something and that food creates a reaction in your body that makes you fat and increases body fat stores, what have you gained? The bottom line is getting rid of body fat. My own research and others have demonstrated that if you eat carbohydrates, you will increase the production of fat and the storage of fat. What difference is there between the fat hanging off a steak and the fat hanging off your beltline? The difference is the fat hanging off your belt line is part of your body and it will be intimately involved in creating problems in your arteries. So you can eat all of the fat in the world, as long as you don't have body fat. This is what I am going to demonstrate. If you lose body fat regardless of what you eat, everything improves.

I'm looking at this from the point of view of a physician and through the eyes of my patients. When I have instructed them to avoid fat and increase their complex carbohydrates, I have encouraged them to store fat on their bodies. As a consequence, all of the things I tried to improve, got worse. I would eventually have my patient on several pills to control blood pressure, cholesterol, and blood sugar. When I knew in my heart that 30 lbs. of weight loss would cure all of these problems and make the pills unnecessary. Since I am looking at obesity and weight loss from a physicians perspective, there are some blood chemistries that I need to explain to you, before I get into the specific examples of how this works and how it makes you healthier.

High cholesterol, high blood pressure, obesity and diabetes have consumed most of my time in the last twenty years. I've been trying to manage these in my patients so they would avoid heart disease, kidney disease and general circulation problems. From this point of view, I want to discuss some terms that I will be referring to in the forthcoming chapters. Let's start with cholesterol. Cholesterol, interestingly enough, is not fat, but is a sterol. Cholesterol is a waxy solid alcohol, which is soapy in appearance and is found in animal fat. Every cell in your body needs cholesterol. More than 90% of the cholesterol in your body is within the cell structure. It is vital for cell wall production, for the production of steroid hormones such as estrogen and testosterone as well as cortisone. If you didn't have enough cholesterol in your body, you would die. That is exactly why your body manufactures it. If you reduce your cholesterol intake, your body will frantically increase its production. Most of this production is from the liver. One of the most potent stimulants of cholesterol production in the liver is INSULIN. Insulin is stimulated into the blood by carbohydrates. Fat causes almost no insulin stimulation. So if you want to INCREASE your production of cholesterol, eat pure carbohydrates. Cholesterol is also vital in the absorption of certain essential fat soluble vitamins, such as vitamin A, D and K. Cholesterol is also vital to the skin, for natural bone growth and to maintaining bone structure. Without cholesterol you could not make vitamin D which is essential in calcium absorption to prevent osteoporosis. So far it sounds like really good stuff, so why are we cholesterol phobic?

Having too much of the WRONG cholesterol in your blood will increase your risk of clogging your arteries and heart disease. But the key is the WRONG kind of cholesterol. The cholesterol itself is not the problem. The problem is what carries the cholesterol in your blood.

LDL AND HDL

There are proteins, called lipoproteins that carry cholesterol. To name a few, LDL - low density lipoprotein, HDL - high density lipoprotein, VLDL - very low density lipoprotein and at least five or six others that go into giving you your total cholesterol. The total cholesterol is meaningless unless you know how much LDL and HDL you have. To simplify matters, we are going to speak of LDL and HDL since they are the predominant ones that we can measure in your blood. LDL cholesterol is the form of most of our cholesterol. The LDL lipoprotein grabs the cholesterol and brings it to its destination. LDL cholesterol's job is to transport cholesterol to the organs so that the organs can use the cholesterol for their structure and function. LDL is a taxicab to bring cholesterol from the liver and intestinal circulation to the organs. The problem appears to be, that substances can alter LDL cholesterol, while it's in the arteries on its way to the organs. That altered protein can be deposited in the arteries. Several things need to happen for this to occur. I will discuss them in detail when we talk about the anatomy of a clogged artery in future chapters. For now, it is important to know that a high LDL cholesterol, especially above 130 mg/dl is thought to increase your risk of heart disease. But that number by itself is not adequate to access your cardiac risk.

The next important type of cholesterol is HDL cholesterol. HDL is denser than LDL thus the high density lipoprotein label. HDL cholesterol is known as the *good* cholesterol because when you have plenty of HDL cholesterol it protects you from LDL cholesterol. How does it do this? HDL cholesterol causes what we call REVERSE CHOLESTEROL TRANSPORT. This means that instead of like LDL bringing cholesterol TO the organs, HDL cholesterol flows through the arteries collecting fat and triglycerides FROM the arteries and brings them back to the liver.

An analogy can be made to a snowstorm. When there is a heavy snowstorm, all the roads and arteries of the city get clogged with snow. This would be similar to the LDL cholesterol transporting cholesterol through the arteries. The snow plows come out and clean the streets and arteries of the city. This is the HDL cholesterol, it will undo what the LDL cholesterol tried to accomplish. That is, unclog the arteries. This is called anti-atherogenic. Atherosclerosis is the clogging and blocking of your arteries. Anti-atherogenic is just the opposite. HDL cholesterol is anti-atherogenic. HDL cholesterol also prevents LDL cholesterol from being oxidized. When you oxidize something you change its chemical structure. When the chemical structure of LDL cholesterol is oxidized in the artery by free radicals, which are free oxygen molecules with missing electrons, the LDL structure is changed. This signals the immune system, the white blood cells, to engulf or eat the LDL cholesterol. LDL cholesterol that has been eaten by a white blood cell is called a FOAM cell. These foam cells then are attracted to areas of the artery that are damaged by stress and blood pressure, created by cigarettes and other toxins, and can accumulate in that spot and create the beginnings of a blockage. There will be more on this in The Anatomy of a Clogged Artery.

DETERMINING YOUR GOOD VS. BAD CHOLESTEROL

So how do I know if my cholesterol is good or bad? The best way to tell if you're okay from the cholesterol viewpoint is a ratio. Take your total amount of cholesterol and divide it by your HDL cholesterol. If this number is less than 4.0, you do not have an increased risk of heart disease based on your cholesterol. If your ratio of total cholesterol divided by your HDL cholesterol is greater than 4.0, then you are at risk from your cholesterol.

Another ratio that is used is to compare your LDL cholesterol to your HDL cholesterol. If you divide your LDL cholesterol by your HDL cholesterol, your number should be 3.0 or less. If it is above 3.0, you are at increased risk. If it is below 3.0 you are not at risk. This is really why there has been such confusion over the past 20 years about cholesterol. A person with a cholesterol of 300 who has an HDL cholesterol of 100, has a ratio of 3.0 of total cholesterol to HDL. That 300 cholesterol is not risky. The reason is that HDL cholesterol acts like a scavenger and takes any fat that is laid down in the vessel and brings it back to the liver, where the liver disposes of the cholesterol through the bowel and out with the bowel movements. So HDL cholesterol will cleanse your arteries and that cholesterol will end up in your toilet bowl with your bowel movement.

An interesting study was done in 1989 by Badimon et al. They fed cholesterol and animal fat to rabbits. This caused fatty streaking or deposits to occur in the aorta or the large major blood vessel in the rabbits. They infused HDL protein and found the fatty streaks disappear . They showed regression of plaque by HDL cholesterol.[1] This was also confirmed by the same investigators as published in The Journal of Clinical Investigation.[2] Anything that INCREASES HDL cholesterol has been found to DECREASE coronary artery disease. Carbohydrates DECREASE HDL cholesterol. Fat and protein intake INCREASE HDL cholesterol. I have demonstrated this in hundreds of patients and I will share the data in future chapters. So when we're concerned about cholesterol, we want to know what our HDL cholesterol is in proportion to the total cholesterol, and what our HDL cholesterol is in proportion to our LDL cholesterol. If our diet makes these worse, we're doing the wrong thing. If our diet makes these better, it's been proven that you will reduce your risk of heart disease. Things we can do to increase our HDL cholesterol, which we want to do, is to lose body fat, quit smoking, reduce carbohydrate intake, and begin or continue to exercise daily.

Triglycerides have been a mystery over the years. Triglyceride levels are usually always elevated in diabetics and in people who are overweight. Triglycerides are the way fats get transported through the body. Usually fat is stored as triglyceride. Triglycerides are a sign of excessive carbohydrate intake and sugar conversion to fat. You're turning sugar into fat when you have high triglycerides. A triglyceride is a glycerol molecule with three fatty acids attached to it. There has been confusion whether triglycerides directly correlate with heart disease. Recent studies show that if your triglyceride level is above 100, you have an increased risk of heart disease and heart attack. The more carbohydrates you eat, the higher your triglyceride goes. A study was published in the Journal of the American Medical Association by Knopp RH. et al[3]. Knopp and Associates evaluated dietary fat restriction and the effect on HDL cholesterol and triglycerides. They took four different diets varying in their fat intake. The first diet group contained 30% of the total diet as fat calories. Group 2 ate 26% of their total calories as fat, Group 3 - 22% fat and Group 4 - 18% of their total calories as fat. The four diets contained 300 mgs of cholesterol, 200 mgs of cholesterol, 100 mgs of cholesterol and 100 mgs of cholesterol mg/dl, respectively. The study addressed two main issues: does greater restriction of fat intake obtain greater LDL lowering after one year and does lipoprotein response differ between dietary regimens?

First order of business was bodyweight. There was no increased weight loss with fat restriction. As the dieters reduced their fat intake, the triglyceride levels elevated. The lower fat increased triglyceride levels and decreased HDL cholesterol levels. This suggested a conversion of cholesterol to a more unfavorable lipid profile containing more of the damaging LDL cholesterol and greater atherogenic properties. The more fat restriction, the more reduction in the HDL cholesterol, the worse these numbers became. HDL's were lower at 18% fat than they were at 30% fat. This has to tell us something. When we restrict fat and eat more carbohydrates our liver makes the wrong kinds of cholesterol.

I took this a step further and did just the opposite. I fed people a low-fat, high carbohydrate diet for three months. I measured their total cholesterol, HDL cholesterol, LDL cholesterol, and triglycerides. I then put these same people on a low carbohydrate, high fat diet and measured the same parameters. When they ate less carbohydrates and more fat, the average HDL cholesterol increased by over 40%. Everyone's HDL cholesterol improved and their total cholesterol/HDL ratio improved . Their LDL cholesterol's did not substantially or significantly elevate and their LDL cholesterol/HDL cholesterol also improved on a low carbohydrate, higher fat and protein diet . My patients were not as excited about this as they were about an average of 20 -25 lbs. of weight loss. They also explained to me that they never felt better, had more energy and most of their gastrointestinal complaints such as indigestion and increased gas disappeared. Twenty-five pounds of fat loss can really improve your body. It is shocking to me how easy this is by doing the total opposite of what we have always been told to do. But every number improves.

DIABETES

Diabetes is another disease that improves with a low carbohydrate diet. Let me just spend some time on the nomenclature of diabetes which I will be referring to, so that you understand how this diet improves a diabetics outcome. Diabetes and obesity are extremely close cousins. There are two types of diabetes. One is what we use to call *Juvenile Onset* because it usually occurred in younger people. They develop an inflammatory reaction in their pancreas and destroy the beta cell of the pancreas so that no insulin is produced. If these people do not get insulin, they will die within months. The striking thing about insulin dependent diabetics are that they are thin. Probably because of the depletion of insulin in their body. They don't have any, they need to inject it.

More than 90% of diabetics are the second type of diabetics called *Adult Onset Diabetic*. The nomenclature has changed to non insulin dependent diabetes because of the fact that some younger people can get this type of diabetes and some older people can get the insulin dependent type. But the vast majority of people who have adult onset diabetes are over 40 years old and are overweight. In my opinion, the only difference between an overweight person and an overweight diabetic, is the fact that the diabetic does not have enough insulin sensitivity to keep his blood sugar down. Everything about these two metabolisms are the same and we can use this in our study of obesity concomitantly for the treatment of our diabetic.

Let's concentrate on the overweight adult onset diabetic. This person makes plenty of insulin. Most of the time if you were to draw an insulin level on a diabetic and compare it to a non-diabetic of the same age, the diabetic would have more insulin in his/her blood than the non-diabetic. How could this be? Insulin brings the blood sugar down. As it turns out, the diabetics insulin doesn't work properly. They have resistance to their own insulin or INSULIN INSENSITIVITY.

The way this works is that when you eat a meal with carbohydrates, the carbohydrates are broken down in your intestines to a simple form of sugar called *glucose*. Glucose will then come into your blood. When the blood sugar level rises, after carbohydrate ingestion, a signal goes off to tell your pancreas to release insulin. Insulin will then allow the sugar to enter your cell. Whether it be a muscle cell, a brain cell, a heart cell or a liver cell. The cell is a little fortress. It will not let anything in, unless there is a password. INSULIN is the password for sugar to get into the cell. Insulin is the doorman, the cell is the apartment building and glucose is the visitor. But insulin needs to be recognized by the cell. There are certain receiving areas on the cell for insulin. They are called *insulin receptors*. If you don't have insulin receptors working properly, the insulin will not be recognized and the cell will not allow sugar to enter it. This is the problem with adult onset diabetics. They have poorly working insulin receptors. As it turns out, increased body fat reduces insulin receptor activity. Losing body fat improves insulin receptors. Remember, there's plenty of insulin but nowhere for the insulin to work. So the blood sugar stays high. By losing body fat, the insulin receptors revive and work better so that the blood sugar comes down. This is the exact problem with obesity. Even though the blood sugar may be maintained normal in an obese non diabetic, their insulin is resistant. Body fat is creating a problem with the receptor on the cell, so that insulin is not working properly. Carbohydrates stimulate more and more insulin. Since you have an unlimited ability to make insulin, you will make as much insulin as you need, to get the blood sugar out of the blood within an hour of eating. If the cells won't receive it because you are overweight and your insulin receptors are not working properly, insulin will turn the sugar into fat called *triglycerides* and store it in the fat warehouse which is usually around our belt. So, unlike the diabetic who will store alot of his sugar as triglycerides and fat but still cannot get the sugar down to normal levels, the obese non diabetic will store ALL the carbohydrates as fat and triglycerides. If you get the insulin out of your blood by not eating carbohydrates, you shut off this mechanism and start to lose body fat instead of gaining it. It's just the opposite of what we've been told. FAT does not cause body fat. CARBOHYDRATES cause body fat. Eating fat makes you <u>lose</u> body fat, eating carbohydrates makes you <u>gain</u> body fat, and it all has to do with that powerful hormone, INSULIN and its actions in the body.

In diabetes, 75% of our diabetics die of heart disease. So we tell our diabetics not to eat fat because we're afraid their cholesterol will be elevated. But we're telling them to eat the one thing they cannot handle, carbohydrates, or sugar. So they eat 60 to 70, sometimes 85% of their calories as carbohydrates and they have no place to put the sugar other than to make it into triglycerides and to store it as fat. No wonder they get worse from all of our advice. In addition, I've shown before, that increasing carbohydrate ingestion will reduce the HDL cholesterol and increase the circulating triglyceride level. This is the OPPOSITE of what you want. Remember, you want more snow plows, not less snow plows. You want to clean out the arteries. So you want HIGHER HDL levels. If you restrict carbohydrates and eat more fat and protein, you will increase your HDL cholesterol and improve your arteries. Isn't it amazing how wrong we are with our current thinking?

GLYCO-HEMOGLOBIN A1C

The other important aspect of diabetes care is to follow how well someones blood sugar is controlled. The complications of diabetes which include blindness, heart disease, stroke, kidney failure and abnormality of the peripheral nerves, called Peripheral Neuropathy is directly related to the blood sugar control. If your blood sugar is perfect, you're very unlikely to get complications of diabetes. If your blood sugar is poorly controlled, you have a great deal of problems in store for you down the road.

The one breakthrough in diabetes care which has been able to help us determine who is controlled and who is not controlled is called the Glyco Hemoglobin (Glyco-Hemoglobin A1C). There was an argument among physicians for the last 15 years as to whether tightly controlling the blood sugar had anything to do with avoiding the complications of diabetes. I can remember when I was training in Montefiore Medical Center in the Bronx, New York that some physicians who were experts in diabetes believed that tight control of diabetes was unnecessary. Why put the patient through the hard task of getting their blood sugar down, if it was not going to reduce his or her complications? As long as their symptoms were controllable, that's all we needed to do. Well this turned out to be totally wrong.

The reason it is wrong is because we did not know how to predict whether someone was controlled or not. Taking a blood sample and checking the blood sugar is just a moment in time. It doesn't tell you what the blood sugar is an hour or two hours later. So it is a very poor judge of glycemic control. Which means the control of the blood sugar. Fortunately, there is a better way to predict this now. A glyco hemoglobin is a unique idea. Researchers were smart enough to figure out that if we could find *something* that has been in the blood for three months and measure how saturated that something was with sugar, we could tell how much average sugar there was in the blood over the last three months.

We know that red blood cells travel around in the blood for three months delivering oxygen. They pick up oxygen in the lungs and are pushed around the blood vessels by the blood pressure. They travel throughout the body releasing their oxygen wherever it's needed. After about three months, the red blood cell gets worn down and wrinkled and the spleen will filter these cells out of the circulation and recycle their vitamins and iron. The iron structure that helps red blood cells have their affinity or attraction to oxygen is called hemoglobin. This is an iron and vitamin made substance in the center of the red blood cell. We can measure the saturation of sugar on the hemoglobin molecule of the red blood cells and tell how well your diabetes is controlled.

A non diabetic with normal blood sugars has a glycohemoglobin of between 4 and 5.8%. That means no more than 5.8% of the persons red blood cell hemoglobin is saturated with sugar. If you take a poorly controlled diabetic, he or she can have anywhere from 10 to 13% of the hemoglobin saturated with sugar. Remember, this is a calculation of what the sugar has been for the past three months. Studies show that if you get the glycohemoglobin below 6.4%, you'll greatly reduce the risks and the complications of diabetes. We finally have an objective measurement. For every 1% above normal, there is increased risk of complications. The problem with diabetes and a low fat, high carbohydrate diet is that we are never able to get the glycohemoglobins below 6.4%. Why? Because they are eating carbohydrates and carbohydrates are sugar, and sugar is their problem.

The average glycohemoglobin of my patients on a low carbohydrate diet is less than 5.8%. They are normal. They have non diabetic blood sugars. People criticize the low carbohydrate diet for many reasons. They say it increases your cholesterol because you eat too much fat. Sorry, it's just the opposite, fellas. They say increasing the protein from eating steak and eggs will damage the kidneys. Sorry fellas, it's not the protein that damages your kidneys, it's the blood sugar elevation that damages kidneys, and if you get the blood sugar down, you don't damage the kidneys. And in fact, if your kidneys are normal, there is no affect of protein on your kidneys. This has been shown in several studies, particularly, a German study in 1995. If you get the sugar down to normal, you won't damage your kidneys. You won't get the sugar down unless you stop eating sugar or carbohydrates.

So when I talk about cholesterol, remember,

1. You want higher HDL cholesterol's and you want the ratio of total cholesterol to HDL cholesterol to be lower or less than 4.0.
2. You want the LDL / HDL cholesterol ratio to be less than 3.0 and you want the total triglycerides less than 100.
3. If you're diabetic, you want your glycohemoglobin to be less than 5.8%.

These are the numbers that you should bring to your doctor. These are the numbers that you should try to obtain. Because these are normal numbers. These reduce the risks of diabetes, hypercholesterolemia, heart disease and stroke. If you are not obtaining these numbers, you should question why. Because there are many people who are attaining them by reducing their carbohydrate intake.

I hope you're still with me.

CHAPTER II.

CARBOHYDRATES - THE REAL ENEMY

The key to weight loss is what food does inside our blood. Your intestines will indiscriminately break down food into its elemental components.

There are three macro nutrients:

1) Carbohydrates

2) Protein

3) Fat

Carbohydrates are either *simple* or *chemically complex* sugars. By the time the intestines breaks down the chemical bonds in a carbohydrate, sugar or glucose will be absorbed into the blood. Once the sugar level starts to rise in the blood after a carbohydrate meal, a signal goes off to instruct your pancreas to release INSULIN. Insulin's job is to remove the sugar from your blood to distribute it to the cells. After the cells are satisfied by taking up sugar and making adenosine triphosphate (ATP) for their function, the rest of the carbohydrates are converted to triglycerides and stored as fat. This is the KEY to the whole diet. INSULIN is the problem. Insulin is the storage hormone. It stores fat, it makes fat from sugar and it does not allow the body to utilize fat as an energy source. This means that the fat you have stored will not be used during your exercise. It is locked in the warehouse and it will not be removed during the time that insulin is in your blood. So if you eat things that bring insulin into your blood, you will not lose weight. That's why the high carbohydrate diet fails. It fails because it does not take into consideration the hormonal changes within the blood after a meal.

The theory for weight loss with the LOW FAT, HIGH COMPLEX CARBOHYDRATE diet is based on the calorie theory. A calorie is the amount of energy required to raise the temperature of one kilogram of water, one degree centigrade. What this has to do with our metabolism totally escapes me. But this is what our entire nutritional recommendations are currently based on. If you eat calories that stimulate a hormone that makes fat, you're not going to lose fat and that's what carbohydrates do. If you don't have insulin in your blood, your body is then free to utilize fat as its energy. Fat will be converted to sugar and will supply energy to the cells. Because this is a very inefficient process and takes alot of work from the body, it requires alot of fat. So that your body fat will be utilized and you will lose weight.

There is another hormone responsible for this called *Glucagon*. Glucagon is the opposite of insulin. Insulin is secreted by your pancreas when the sugar level starts to rise. Glucagon on the other hand, is secreted by the pancreas when your sugar level starts to fall. Your body likes to maintain a certain range of sugar between 70 and 100. When it starts to drop down toward 70 and you don't replenish the sugar stores by eating carbohydrates, glucagon is released to take fat and protein and convert it into sugar. It also reduces fat production and increases fat breakdown. It takes the warehouse of fat we have on our body and turns it into energy. This difference is the key to success. You will lose weight if you don't eat carbohydrates. If you eat more fat and protein, you will be successful. The process of converting protein and triglycerides (glycerol) into glucose (sugar) is called gluconeogenesis. The creation of new glucose from protein and triglyceride. Restricting carbohydrates causes the body to use protein and fat for energy.

LOW FAT DIET - MY WORST ENEMY

This has been demonstrated to me in the tens of thousands of patients that I have taken care of with obesity over the past twenty years. But it really struck home when I found my own situation getting worse despite my own best advice. For the first fifteen years of my medical practice, I adhered to the low-fat, high complex carbohydrate theory on healthful eating. I wouldn't eat meat, cheese, or eggs if my life depended on it. I ate breakfast cereal , fruits, vegetables, potatoes, bread , rice and pasta. I never had desserts and I exercised vigorously. This worked well, until I turned 40. I was running 15 miles a week and working out 4 days a week at Gold's Gym. My theory was that if I increased my muscle mass, I would increase my metabolism and burn more fat. I was the health police. If my nurses or receptionists were eating fat, I would point out how many grams of fat they were eating and make their lives miserable. My cholesterol had always been 180 with an HDL of 60 and an LDL less than 130, numbers I will explain in detail in the upcoming chapters. However, after the age of 40 despite my low-fat, high carbohydrate diet, I started to gain body fat. The definition of my muscles were hard to discern and most shocking of all, my cholesterol was rising. For the first time, my LDL cholesterol was 141. Something was wrong. But this was exactly what I had observed in my patients over the last fifteen years.

My patients would explain that they did not eat large amounts of calories and avoided fat at all costs. They, however were getting fat and as a consequence, their blood pressure, cholesterol and diabetes were not improving. My explanation was usually that they were not adhering to the low-fat diet and not exercising enough. Until of course, it started happening to me. How could we be wrong? How could all of the experts be traveling down the wrong road? But the great thing about human nature is that if something doesn't work, you eventually stop doing it. I will discuss some of the patients I have cared for that helped open up my eyes to the low-carbohydrate, low insulin secreting diet.

I thank them all for the lessons they have taught me.

THE STORY OF JOE D.

(Joe D. is Dr. Joseph Hickey's father-in-law)

Joe D. is a 70 year old patient who was obese at 5 foot 8 inches tall and 220 lbs. His cholesterol however, was 142. Of some concern to me was an HDL cholesterol of 27 but with an LDL cholesterol well below 130, I felt he had little risk of coronary artery disease. He also had mild hyperglycemia with a fasting blood sugar of 130. It should be less than 110 mg. In 1992 this was borderline diabetes and merely required diet therapy. So we embarked upon a low-fat , cholesterol controlled, high complex carbohydrate diet. His wife, Marie was fanatical about fat restriction. She gave him breakfast cereal, mostly Special K, a banana and sometimes raisins for breakfast with skim milk. Salad with skinless chicken breast for lunch and usually pasta, rice, potatoes and vegetables for dinner with fruit and crackers for dessert. She avoided cheese, meat and eggs religiously. Joe continued to get fatter. His blood pressure was fine, and with the level of cholesterol being 142, I did not feel any other intervention was necessary.

In 1992, Joe started to get chest pain with exertion. This led to angiography. *Angiography* is when we take dye and shoot it into the coronary arteries to see where the blockages are forming. Joe had a 95% blocked right coronary artery and a 40% blocked left anterior descending coronary artery. The three major arteries are the right coronary artery, the left coronary artery and a branch off of the left coronary artery called the circumflex. We attempted to do angioplasty on Joe's right coronary artery, but it was so solidly blocked that they could not open up the artery with the balloon. He had coronary artery bypass surgery as the only alternative because he continued to have chest pain and signs of an impending heart attack. The other arteries in his heart were clear, except for the 40% blockage of the left anterior descending artery. It was felt at that time by the cardiologists that it would take so long for him to block that artery in view of the fact that he was 70 years old, that we would not need to do anything other than cholesterol lowering diet for his remaining blocked artery. He got through coronary bypass surgery successfully, and felt well for the next five years.

During that time, his wife became more fanatical about Joe's avoidance of fat. Again, I monitored his cholesterols religiously and his cholesterol never got above 160. His HDL however, was between 20 and 28. His blood sugars also started to rise, probably because of all of the carbohydrates he was eating and he continued to gain weight. His weight went up to 230 lbs. despite almost total fat restriction. The other thing I noticed about Joe D. was the more he avoided fat, the lower his HDL cholesterol sunk. In 1997, Joe started to get chest pain again. We repeated his cardiac catherization and angiography and found at this point ALL his coronary arteries were now blocked. His bypass graft was still open but the other arteries progressed to severe 95% narrowings in five years. Not only the one that was initially blocked at 40%, but the other clear arteries were blocked. He then had a repeat bypass surgery. At this point, I knew his low-fat, high complex carbohydrate diet was not working.

We totally switched gears. I told him to restrict his carbohydrates to less than 25 grams total a day, and to ignore the fat and protein that he ate. Within three months, Joe D. lost 40 lbs., his cholesterol went from 142 to 180, but his HDL cholesterol went from 27 to 78. His total cholesterol/HDL cholesterol ratio, improved dramatically. Studies show that the most important reading is to have a total cholesterol divided by your HDL at less than the number 4. Prior to our low carbohydrate diet, Joe's cholesterol was 142, HDL of 28 giving him a cholesterol /HDL ratio of 5.0. Then we restricted his carbohydrates to less than 25 grams a day. Currently Joe's total cholesterol of 186 divided by his HDL cholesterol of 78 is 2.4. A dramatic improvement in his overall cholesterol.

Joe was happy that he could now eat eggs, cheese and meat and in the process lost 40 lbs. He went down 3 belt sizes. How could this be? INSULIN. With all of the carbohydrates he was eating, he needed more and more insulin to store the carbohydrates. He ate more carbohydrates than his cells could use, so he stored most of it in the form of triglycerides and fat. He got fatter & fatter and his HDL cholesterol got lower & lower. Insulin is thought to create the blockages in your arteries. When you eat large amounts of carbohydrates because you're trying to avoid fat, the cells of your body get so saturated with sugar, that the receptors on those cells tend to work less efficiently. We call this in medicine *down regulation of the receptor*. The receptors become less efficient at picking up insulin and sugar. So you need more and more insulin to get the cells to respond to sugar. This is called INSULIN RESISTANCE . You've become resistant to your own insulin because of overuse. Because insulin's job is to remove sugar from your blood, and because the cells will no longer accept it unconditionally, insulin then turns the sugar into fat by increasing fat and cholesterol metabolism by your liver. This is how you get fatter from carbohydrates. We reversed the process in Joe D. by taking him off of carbohydrates. He now eats sausage or bacon with eggs for breakfast, he has chicken or tuna salad for lunch in a large portion with plenty of regular mayonnaise and he eats beef, pork or chicken with broccoli or other green vegetables for dinner. There is no calorie counting because we're relying on the glucagon that he is secreting to reduce his fat stores. We are restricting the insulin he makes, which reduces his fat storage.

THE STORY OF MARIE D.

The next example of dramatic reversal of cholesterol and body weight came with Joe D.'s wife, Marie D. (my mother-in-law). When Marie saw the reversal in Joe D.'s cholesterol, HDL and body fat (40 lbs) with a low carbohydrate diet, she was distressed. "The man had two bypass surgeries in 5 years. His HDL continued to fall. I was killing him with a low fat diet." She was right. Unfortunately, it was my advice to them based on what I had been taught from my reading of the medical literature. I was not stupid enough to put Joe D. back on a low fat diet a third time, Thank God.

SYSTOLIC & DIASTOLIC BLOOD PRESSURES

Marie had her own health problems. Her blood pressure was always resistant to my efforts. The systolic blood pressure was always around 165 to 180 despite multiple medications. SYSTOLIC blood pressure is the top number of a blood pressure. The DIASTOLIC blood pressure is the bottom number. Your systolic blood pressure should be 120 (top number). Your diastolic blood pressure should be 80 or less. SYSTOLIC means the pressure created when your heart is contracting and pumping the blood into your aorta and arteries. The reason it is higher than the bottom number is because the heart is violently contracting and pushing blood through your arteries to circulate oxygen and nutrients throughout your body. Without this forcible pumping pressure (systolic), you could not circulate oxygen and you would die. Think of it like this - you need a good water pressure in your pipes to get hot water to your upstairs bathroom. Without that force in your pipes, you could not take a shower upstairs. But if the pressure is TOO high in the pipes, they will eventually weaken and burst. Hopefully this occurs AFTER you sell your house.

If you do not have a well working heart pump, you cannot make a good systolic pressure, and you will not get blood and oxygen to your upstairs bathroom, YOUR BRAIN. When you stand up or sit up, gravity pulls the fluid and blood down towards your feet. Your heart and arteries must then push the blood up hill toward your head to maintain blood flow. If the pressure is TOO LOW (systolic pressure below 80, and for elderly below 100) you will get dizzy and pass out. We see this when we give blood pressure medicines that drop your top number (systolic blood pressure) too low. This is called HYPOTENSION. The opposite of HYPERTENSION. If you stand up and you get dizzy or lightheaded, have your blood pressure checked while you are standing. This is when you need some pressure in your arteries. If you are on blood pressure medicines, and you stand up and get light headed, your doctor needs to change your dose, or type of blood pressure medication.

The *DIASTOLIC* blood pressure is the bottom number on your blood pressure reading. During diastole, your heart is not pumping. This is between heartbeats. Your heart is filling up with blood during this period. So it can pump or push out the blood to create a systolic pressure with the next heartbeat. Diastole or diastolic blood pressure is in between heart beats or while the heart muscle is resting and recovering. So the diastolic or lower number is more related to the tension created and maintained in your arteries between heartbeats. When your heart beats and pushes blood into the arteries, the arteries relax and dilate, accepting the pressure from the heart. The relaxation of this rubber-like muscular arterial tube will then absorb the pressure from your heartbeat and cushion the pressure. This property of the artery is called *compliance*. It complies with the systolic pressure and relaxes, thereby absorbing some of the pressure. Your artery can do this because it is a tube made up of collagen and smooth, soft muscle. If your arteries become stiff and hardened (the Greek word for this is atherosclerosis, athero means gruel, sclerosis means hard or stiff), they will not relax and comply with the pressure created by your heart. Because they are hardened and stiff, the blood pressure goes up to high levels.

When your heart is relaxing and the force inside your arteries starts to fall, the arterial smooth muscle will contract and make the tube smaller in diameter. This will maintain some pressure in your arteries between heart beats. You need this pressure to be maintained in your arteries in between heartbeats to continue to circulate your blood. If it dropped to zero in between heartbeats, you would not circulate blood during that period. In other words, if you have two upstairs showers, and your visitor is taking a shower, in order for you to be able to shower at the same time, you will need enough pressure in your pipes. Without this pressure, the water will not flow to either shower when both are turned on.

It is the same concept with your circulation. In between heartbeats, your arterial smooth muscle must contract to maintain pressure during diastole or the resting phase. This is your bottom number or diastolic blood pressure. If your lower or diastolic blood pressure drops below 50 in between heartbeats, you will also get dizzy and pass out due to the lack of oxygen circulation to the brain. This process of relaxation of the artery and constriction of the artery must occur with each heartbeat to maintain your pressure at 120/80. The smooth muscle inside your artery is responsible for this amazing adaptation. If the arterial muscle is stiff and hardened, your pressure for systole will be high at 180 - 200. And when the heart relaxes, the muscle cannot adapt or comply, so the bottom number falls precipitously below 50. This is a sign of atherosclerosis.

A pressure of 180/50 is the type you would see in elderly people. Through wear and tear on their artery, they have become hardened and non compliant. This is difficult to treat with medications because when you lower the systolic blood pressure to below 140 with medicines, you also lower the bottom pressure below 50. The person will then get dizzy or pass out when he or she stands up. This was described by the great European physician Sir William Osler in the 19th Century. He would measure the blood pressure and record the top number, or systolic BP, say for example, 160 mm/mercury. Then he would pump the cuff to say 200. At 200 (above the persons systolic BP) there should be no further blood flow through that artery. The artery will then empty and collapse if it is compliant and not hardened. If Dr. Osler put the blood pressure cuff on his patients arm just above the elbow, and pumped the cuff up above that persons pressure, the pulse he felt in the wrist should disappear and the artery should collapse. You will no longer feel the pulse or the artery in the wrist. But if the person has Atherosclerosis, or hardening of the arteries, when the cuff is pumped up above the pressure, the pulse will disappear in the wrist, but, you will still feel the artery. It feels like a small stiff tube in the wrist and does not collapse. This is called Osler's sign. I used this for years to teach my medical students at New York Medical College how to assess the state of one's arteries. If they have Osler's sign, you must be careful trying to lower that top number or the patients will be passing out all over town.

People who have both numbers elevated, 180/110, probably have too much size (hypertrophy) or thickness to the arterial smooth muscle. Their arteries have become muscle bound and inflexible. The things that make your arterial smooth muscle too thick, non compliant and muscle bound are hypertension, cigarette smoking, obesity and too much insulin in your blood. Insulin stimulates the smooth muscle in your arteries to grow bigger and stiffens artery muscles. Obesity and insulin do this better than anything else I know. If you do not lose body fat and reduce the insulin level in your arteries, there will come a point where losing weight will not help your blood pressure. The arterial muscle becomes so thick and enlarged that the process is now irreversible. Even losing body fat at that point does not bring down the blood pressure. The hypertension is fixed in and very difficult to control even with medicines.

For years we were taught that the bottom blood pressure or diastolic pressure was the most important to control. If the heart has to pump into an artery with a diastolic pressure of 110 mm/mercury, it has to work harder than if the blood pressure is 70 mm/mercury. The harder the heart has to pump, the faster it will enlarge and eventually become weak. Soon it will be unable to make any blood pressure, and you will need a new heart, if you can get one.

Studies now show that the systolic or top pressure is actually more risky than the diastolic. The risk of heart attack and especially stroke seems correlated most with the systolic pressure. A systolic pressure above 130 increases your risk of heart attack and stroke tremendously. A diastolic pressure above 85 mm/mercury increases your chance of weakening or dilating your heart. You will then develop *cardiomyopathy* and *congestive heart failure*. Since the pump does not pump anymore, the pump backs up. The fluid in your blood then backs up into your lungs and fills the air space with water. The end result is you cannot breath and you will continuously cough to try and dispel the water from your lungs. You are drowning. You then need water pills, (diuretics) to remove water from your lungs. It seems to me that both of these pressures need controlling. But if the pressure gets fixed in because of too much thickness to your artery wall, or as Dr. Osler described, the artery gets hardened, it is then very difficult to fix the blood pressure with pills. We can help with pills, but we cannot fix the blood pressure. It is an abnormal anatomical and physiological state of your arteries. In my 20 years of medicine, nothing contributes more to this hypertension, than cigarettes, obesity and too much insulin stimulation by carbohydrates.

Now, back to my mother-in-law. Marie D. had BOTH blood pressures elevated at 180-190 over 105 mm/mercury. Marie is 5 feet 7 inches. At the time of her marriage to Joe D., her weight was 110 lbs. At age 60, Marie's weight was 150 lbs. (sorry, Mom!). I made her a Fat Free Fanatic after Joe D.'s first heart surgery. We both became CHOLESTEROL and FAT PHOBIC. Marie was steadily gaining weight and her blood pressure was resistant. She ate pasta, pasta, and more pasta. We followed the recommendations by the Hypertension Control and Detection Panel, and the

National Committee of Blood Pressure Experts which was to start with salt restriction.

We restricted Marie's salt, her pressure got worse. Subsequently, studies are beginning to show that for most people, salt restriction is dangerous. Less than 30% of people with high blood pressure will improve their pressure with salt restriction. The restriction in salt is not without consequences. Alderman MH, et al reported a study in the medical journal The Lancet, this year.[4] The authors of this study examined the relationship of salt intake to cardiovascular disease and to all-cause mortality.

They studied 20,000 men and women between the ages of 25 and 75 years old. Some of these people restricted salt, others did not. Of this group, approximately 10,000 of these people were free of any cardiovascular disease. Analysis of this study indicates that sodium or salt intake was INVERSELY associated with both all-cause mortality and cardiovascular death. Inversely associated means the opposite direction. The more salt you restricted, the more likely you were to die. The more salt you ate, the less likely you would have a heart attack. Sorry mom, I was wrong again. You can go back to the salt shaker!

The exception to this seems to be African-Americans. African-Americans high blood pressure seem to be the blood pressure that is salt sensitive. Restricting salt and the use of salt and water losing pills (diuretics) actually help these blood pressures. My theory on this is that Africa, being mostly below the Equator and a very hot, dry place, requires its inhabitants to be able to have tremendous salt and water retaining abilities to be able to survive periods of time without salt and water. Salt water is what helps maintain our blood pressure. It is what our heart pumps around to fill our cardiovascular system. When we forced and kidnapped Africans to come here to America by means of that unspeakably inhuman slavery, we forced them to adapt to a climate that does not require as much salt retaining ability. In addition, our diet is the highest in salt intake in the world. That environment and diet adaptation obviously takes more than 300 years. Couple that with the prejudice and indignity that African-Americans have had to endure, it's no wonder their hypertension is different than white Americans hypertension. So in my African-American patients, I will try salt restriction and it usually helps.

The other exceptions to salt restriction are people with weakly pumping hearts (Congestive Heart Failure), and people with poorly functioning kidneys (Renal Failure). The weak heart cannot pump salt and water around, so you must constrict it. The weak kidney cannot filter salt and water, it will accumulate in the body and drown us. So heart failure and kidney failure patients need to lighten or restrict salt load. Marie D. went back on salt and her blood pressure actually improved a little to 160-170/100.

The next recommendation of the panel of experts was to use a beta blocker. Beta blockers block the beta receptor on our heart and arteries. The beta receptor receives adrenaline which will increase the force of our hearts contraction and constrict our arteries. Adrenaline will raise our blood pressure. A beta blocker will block that receptor and nullify the actions of adrenaline. This did not lower Marie's blood pressure. It did however, make her tired and lethargic.

Next, I tried ace-inhibitors which block a chemical that causes our arteries to constrict. Ace inhibitors block angiotension converting enzyme. Angiotension I is lying inert in our lungs. When it is activated by angiotension converting enzyme, it then spreads to our blood vessels and constricts them. This is a fail-safe mechanism that we have for when we are losing fluid from dehydration or losing blood from hemorrhaging. Angiotension will keep our blood pressure high so that we do not go into shock. It will buy us some time until we drink some fluids (salt water), or stop the bleeding. People with high blood pressure sometimes make too much angiotension. We can block this with an ace-inhibitor. This is an especially important drug to use in a diabetic with hypertension. Ace inhibitors can save a diabetic's kidneys. It is also crucial to use in people with congestive heart failure. It relaxes the artery smooth muscle and reduces the tension in the artery against which the heart has to pump. This will reduce the enlargement and failure of the heart. If you have congestive heart failure or hypertension with diabetes, and you are not on an ace-inhibitor, your doctor owes you an explanation.

Unfortunately, the ace-inhibitor did not improve Marie D.'s blood pressure. It did however, cause a chronic cough. Since ace-inhibitors inhibit angiotension, which is stored in your lungs, it sometimes causes a spill over of chemicals called *kinins*. These kinins cause a harmless, but persistent pestering dry cough. It is totally reversible in 2 weeks after stopping the medicine. Sorry Mom, off with the ace-inhibitor.

Next we tried the newer calcium channel blocker - Procardia. Finally, we got some response. Marie's blood pressure came down to 150/70. Not optimal for risk factor reduction, but improved. This lasted 6 months. Then Marie's feet began to swell. This is a known side effect to all calcium blockers. They relax the veins and arteries in your circulation and cause fluid to leak out of your veins. Your feet and ankles then swell.

"Joey, (Dr. Hickey), I can't get my shoes on," she clamored.

"Mom, you will have to get bigger shoes. I finally found something that will bring your blood pressure down a little," I explained.

She bought that for awhile until her dentist started to notice that her gums were growing over her teeth. She was developing gum hypertrophy, or growth from the calcium blocker. Uh-oh, we better stop the medicine. In one month, the swelling in her gums and the swelling in her feet disappeared.

At the same time, I was having trouble with Marie's cholesterol. It was not high, but she also had no HDL.

Marie and Joe D. were on the lowest fat diet in history. I saw to that. Marie's blood pressure was not controllable. Her cholesterol was also TERRIBLE. Her total was 200, but her HDL was only 25. That gave her a total cholesterol (200) HDL cholesterol (25) ratio of 200/25 = 8. It should be less than 4. My next move, of course was a cholesterol pill. I started with Mevacor, then Pravachol, then Lescol, then Zocor and finally Lipitor. Her cholesterol numbers did improve. Her total cholesterol came down to 170 mg. Her HDL went up to 39 mg. and LDL was a comfortable 87 mg. Your LDL should be less than 130 mg. IF YOU HAVE HEART DISEASE OR DIABETES, YOUR LDL SHOULD BE LESS THAN 100 MG. So, I felt a little better about myself, even if I could not control her blood pressure after every medicine in the book. I was concerned however, about her Total cholesterol/HDL ratio. It had improved from 8 to 6.7, but remember Joe D. had two different bypass surgeries on his arteries and his ratio at that time was 5.0 (142/28 = 5).

Finally Marie exclaimed, "Joey, if your father-in-law lost 40 lbs. and more than tripled his HDL, shouldn't I be on this low carbohydrate diet?" As you can see, I'm no genius. If she wasn't my mother-in-law, she would have dumped me as a physician long ago.

But just to remain my academic self, I had her get a fasting insulin level. I was beginning to realize that Insulin Resistance was probably behind most of the obesity and hypertension I was treating. Your fasting insulin level should be less than 10. Marie's was a shocking 95! She was the lowfat, high complex carbohydrate fanatic, thanks to me, and I was killing her too. I immediately took her off of carbohydrates, restricting her to less than 30 grams a day. I did not limit anything else.

In three months of carbohydrate restriction, Marie lost 20 lbs. Her weight was now 130. Her cholesterol dramatically improved. Her total cholesterol did go up from 170 to 198, but her HDL also went up from 39 to 52. Her LDL went down to 107. Her Total Cholesterol to HDL ratio went from 6.7 to 3.6. Finally, it is BELOW 4.0. And you guessed it - her blood pressure is now 140/70.

Hopefully, with time, the smooth muscle hypertrophy and enlargement in her arteries that was caused by insulin will shrink and her blood pressure will come down further. She went back to her old shoes, also.

This points out, pure and simple, carbohydrates induce *hyperinsulinism.* It also points out the effect of insulin on blood pressure and HDL cholesterol.

ALL IN THE FAMILY

Now, after Marie's sister Aunt Gloria saw the weight loss Marie obtained, she immediately said, "Give me Joey's diet." Gloria is 5 feet 4 inches tall. She was 113 lbs when she got married. In the fall of 1997, Aunt Glo was 169 lbs. (sorry, Aunt Glo). After 3 months of Joey's (Dr. Hickey) diet, she is down to 138 lbs. (look'in fine now, Aunt Glo).

To complete this family tree, I must tell you about Frank D. Ironically, Joe D. and Frank D. are brothers. Marie D. and Gloria D. are sisters. Marie married Joe, and Gloria married Frank. Two brothers married two sisters.

After my experience with Joe D., Marie D. and with Aunt Glo's success, Uncle Frank decided to join the bandwagon. Uncle Frank is 5 feet 6 inches tall. He weighed 150 lbs. at the time of his marriage, over 30 years ago. He now weighed 185 lbs. After 3 months on carbohydrate restriction, he is now down to 156. A dramatic improvement.

Now, Frank is 67 years old. His brother, Joe D. had his first sign of heart trouble at age 70 years. So I was at least curious to see if 20 years of low-fat diet had ruined Frank's arteries also. He underwent a stress test, which is an exercise treadmill test, while you are hooked up to an ECG (electrocardiogram). With a doctor at your side monitoring your electrical heart response to exercise, he or she can tell if you have a blockage in your artery and even which artery is blocked. Frank did not last 5 minutes on the treadmill when I stopped it. His ECG response showed definite trouble. I took him immediately to Dr. James Johnston, interventional cardiologist par excellent. He had a coronary angiogram that showed multiple critical blockages. Especially, a 90% blocked Left Anterior Descending Artery (LAD) with ulcerated plaque. If the plaque is ulcerated, it is ready to form a blood clot and close completely. The LAD artery, we doctors call the "Widow Maker", because it supplies most of the pumping area of the heart.

Uncle Frank had successful coronary bypass surgery by the brilliant, Dr. David Capallo, at St. Joseph's Hospital in Savannah, Georgia near my office in Hilton Head, S.C.. Uncle Frank is home safe and now on a LOW CARBOHYDRATE DIET.

PLEASE, IF YOU ARE OVER 50 YEARS OLD, ASK YOUR DOCTOR ABOUT A STRESS TEST. IF HE OR SHE TELLS YOU, YOU DON'T NEED ONE, FIND ANOTHER DOCTOR.

THE STORY OF CHERYL M.

The next patient who opened my eyes was Cheryl M. Cheryl is a 32 year old mother of three. She was married at the age of 20 and proceeded having her children. She was 115 lbs at the time of her wedding. At age 32, she was 157 lbs. She would not be seen in a bathing suit, and her weight loss efforts met with failure. She restricted fat and relied upon pasta, rice and complex carbohydrates. After taking her dietary history, we agreed that she had followed all the rules. She was exercising fairly vigorously, but was not getting any results. So we tried the opposite approach. It wasn't hard to convince Cheryl to eat more fat and protein and to restrict carbohydrates because she had done just the opposite for 10 years and had gained 30 lbs. Cheryl began eating eggs and bacon for breakfast without toast. She avoided fruit juices because of their high sugar concentration, she ate cold cuts and cheese for lunch and ate steak and salad for dinner. She had diet jello with whip cream for dessert and that satisfied her sweet tooth. Cheryl lost 40 lbs. in 6 months. She has read all of the reports that low carbohydrate diets create fluid loss but not real fat loss. She scoffs at this. She's happy, has more energy and she's back in a bikini bathing suit. It's hard to tell Cheryl that this is the wrong way to eat.

LENNY C.

The next important observation I made was the case of Lenny C. Lenny was an old high school friend of mine who I have known now for over the 30 years. Lenny's father died while we were still in high school at the age of 45 from a sudden myocardial infarction. His life was taken away tragically at a very early age. Because of this, after I came home from my residency at Montefiore Hospital and Albert Einstein College of Medicine in the Bronx, NY, I immediately had Lenny come in for a cholesterol check.

Not to my surprise, I found Lenny's numbers to be terrible. His cholesterol was over 400 and his triglyceride level was over 1500. His wife and I badgered him for the next 3 - 4 years to reduce fat and rely on a low-fat, high carbohydrate diet. We specified the carbohydrates to be complex carbohydrates including the usual suspects, oatmeal, breakfast cereal, pasta; and we told him to avoid meat, cheese, eggs and saturated fat. Lenny began to get fat on this diet and his cholesterol got worse. In the mid 1980's a breakthrough in cholesterol lowering was put on the market called Mevacor.

We immediately started Lenny on Mevacor and gradually increased him to the maximum dose. His cholesterol improved to 280, his triglycerides came down to 400. However, his HDL cholesterol was still less than 35. HDL cholesterol of less than 35 is an independent risk factor for heart disease. We continued to badger Lenny on his diet and to make sure that he did not take in more than 20% of his calories as fat. Over the next 20 years, Lenny gained 40 lbs. of body fat. He avoided saturated fat as if it were a disease. In 1997, Lenny had a heart attack. On his own, Lenny decided to totally switch gears. If what I was telling him did not work, he was stubborn enough to try just the opposite. Lenny restricted carbohydrates to less than 30 grams a day and ate eggs, meat, cheese and totally disregarded the fat intake. Lenny lost 35 lbs. in four months. His triglycerides went from 350 which we achieved by the newest cholesterol gun, Lipitor, to a sparkling level of 85. His cholesterol went from 280 to 180 and his HDL cholesterol is now above 50. Incredible, but true. Lenny will not go back to a low fat diet.

GETTING THE MESSAGE: PATIENT JOHN D.

At this point , I was getting the message. When John D. came into my office with obesity, hypertension and diabetes, and the usual story that he avoided fats, but was getting fat, I took very little time in deciding to try to convince him to switch gears. Diabetes is a very special case. Diabetes is the inability to process blood sugar. Seventy- five percent of diabetics die of a heart attack or stroke. It is a strong recommendation of the American Heart Association to avoid saturated fat to less than 30% of the total daily calories. In fact, there are some very strong recommendations to reduce your fat to 20% of the total calories when you have diabetes. I followed this recommendation in my patients for 15 years. There is no more frustrating condition to treat than diabetes when you follow a lowfat diet. Diabetics have trouble regulating their blood sugar. You're feeding them carbohydrates. The recommendation is between 50 & 80% of their total calories to be complex carbohydrates. This is all converted to sugar. They can't handle sugar, so the sugar becomes difficult to control. Adult Onset diabetics have plenty of circulating insulin, it just doesn't work to distribute the sugar out of their blood. They are resistant to their own insulin. The standard treatments for diabetes in the adult is weight loss and glucose control. Weight loss is impossible because they have such high insulin levels. Remember that insulin promotes fat storage and fat production by the liver. While avoiding fat, so they don't get heart disease, we're *causing* it by feeding them carbohydrates. We then will start him on medication to further increase his insulin level so that we can bring the blood sugar down. His blood sugar improves, but because of the increased insulin that he is secreting, he gets more obese and more hypertensive. His blood pressure climbs, his cholesterol climbs, his bodyweight climbs, but his sugar is now improved.

Eventually, within 3 - 4 years his blood sugar will start to rise again because he can't make enough insulin to satisfy his now poorly responsive insulin receptors. We then put him on insulin. This further complicates his weight and he continues to get more body fat and it becomes a viscous cycle. The first thing I did with John D., who was already on insulin and 40 lbs overweight with a blood sugar of 300 was to check his C Peptide level. *C peptide* is the tail end of one's own insulin. If he's still making plenty of insulin despite the fact that we're giving him insulin, I can measure it with a C peptide level. This will not detect the insulin he's injecting, but only his endogenously produced insulin.

John was now up to 50 units of injected insulin a day. His C peptide level was above normal which means he was also secreting more than normal amounts of insulin from his pancreas. We were feeding the fire with this low fat, high complex carbohydrate diet. We immediately reversed gears. We had plenty of incentive. He was 30 lbs. overweight, his blood sugar was 300, he was on 50 units of injected insulin, his triglyceride level was 700 and his cholesterol 280 with an HDL cholesterol of 34. We placed John D. on a low carbohydrate diet and restricted carbohydrates to less than 25 grams a day for 3 months, and the usual reversal occurred. He lost 30 lbs., his blood sugar normalized and his cholesterol completely reversed. His triglycerides were less than 150, his cholesterol 200 and his HDL now 70. The most intriguing thing was his blood sugar control. Remember what a glycohemoglobin is? The average sugar reading over the past 3 months. John D.'s glycohemoglobin , despite the fact that he was on 50 units of insulin, was 11%. After 4 months and 30 lbs of fat loss , his glycohemoglobin was 5.9%. We totally reversed his diabetes and made him very happy.

The key to these successes was carbohydrate restriction. Carbohydrates are the gun and insulin is the bullet. By restricting carbohydrates, you restrict the outflow of insulin from the pancreas. Insulin makes you fat, it makes you stay fat and it doesn't let fat get broken down for energy use. By restricting carbohydrates you reduce the insulin that circulates in your blood and you rely more on glucagon which takes fat and turns it into energy. That's why you lose weight, that's why your cholesterol gets better and that's probably why the HDL rises and the LDL cholesterol falls. The bottom line - restrict carbohydrates and you will lose weight. In the process, you will make yourself healthier. This will work for any obese person because they have naturally become resistant to their own insulin. They may or may not eventually become diabetic when their insulin levels fail and their resistance to insulin remains intact. The only way to improve your insulin receptors and your insulin function is to lose body fat. You need to put out the fire and restrict carbohydrates. In my study of nutrition over the past 20 years , many criticisms of the low carbohydrate, higher fat and protein diet have surfaced.

CRITICISM #1:

Higher fat content of the diet will increase the risk of cholesterol.

The previous examples I have just given are just a few examples of the many patients that I have seen do just the opposite. Their cholesterol completely reverses to an improved level. I have over 100 patients who have at least doubled their HDL cholesterol and reduced their total Cholesterol/HDL ratio. Low HDL syndrome or an HDL cholesterol less than 35 is a serious problem and increases the risk of heart disease. A case controlled study of men with angiographically proven coronary artery disease showed that over 1/3 of these men had total cholesterol levels below 200. And of these men 3/4 had HDL cholesterols less than 35. [5]

I see more heart attacks related to low HDL than I do high LDL's. The important thing to remember is that if you increase your HDL cholesterol, you increase the snow plows. You reduce the blockages of the arteries. It may be necessary to use a cholesterol lowering medicines along with a high fat diet. This would hit the cholesterol at both ends. It would increase the HDL to improve the scavenger activity of HDL and thereby cleaning out our arteries and we can reduce the production of LDL cholesterol by the liver. If you use a cholesterol lowering medicine by itself, you may also decrease the HDL production. The LDL or bad cholesterol lowering drugs we call *statins*, are real breakthroughs. Statins are the following: Mevacor, Pravachol, Lipitor, Zocor, Baycol and Lescol. These medicines have dramatically improved cholesterols by reducing the liver's ability to make cholesterol. Remember, insulin stimulates the liver to increase production of cholesterol. Carbohydrates stimulate insulin.

The chemical reaction in the liver that is stimulated, is run by an enzyme (protein) called 3 - hydroxy, 3 - methyl, glutaryl, co enzyme A (HMG - CoA reductase). This enzyme is stimulated by insulin to increase the rate of cholesterol production. This enzyme controls synthesis of cholesterol. The statin medications mentioned above, block the activity of this enzyme so that it cannot efficiently produce cholesterol. You can do this naturally with carbohydrate restriction. When you reduce body fat, a process called lipolysis, you increase HDL. When you increase body fat, a process called lipogenesis, you decrease HDL cholesterol. Nothing creates lipolysis and prevents lipogenesis better than a low-carbohydrate diet. So improve your HDL's and you will improve your risk of coronary disease.

If you have hypertension, body weight is directly related to blood pressure. There is a direct relationship between body weight and the level of blood pressure. Weight loss closely correlates with blood pressure reduction. This effect is independent of dietary sodium restriction. If you lose body fat you improve your blood sugar , if you're a diabetic. Improved blood sugar reduces the complications of diabetes. You have to ask yourself, is a low carbohydrate diet healthy? If you're losing body fat, improving your blood pressure, increasing your HDL cholesterol , reducing your insulin resistance, improving your blood sugar and losing 30 lbs., you tell me.

Table 1 will show improved cholesterol profiles with a low carbohydrate diet. The only instruction I gave to patients was to restrict carbohydrates in their diet to less than 40 grams a day. I did not limit fat or protein intake. I told them to completely ignore the fat contents in the food and to just concentrate on how many grams of carbohydrates they were taking in. Previous to this diet change, they were all following a low fat diet with 30% of their total calories as fat, 60% of their total calories as carbohydrates and 10% of their total calories as protein. Please observe the before and after numbers. Every single person improved their cholesterol/HDL ratio, triglyceride level and total HDL cholesterol and everyone lost weight.

Table 2 shows improved Glycohemoglobin A1C's in diabetics, their weight loss and improvement in their lipid profiles. Their baseline numbers are on a lowfat diet with 30 grams of fat or less as their total calories a day and the second readings are with a low carbohydrate diet with 40 grams or less carbohydrates per day. Note the improvement of the Hemoglobin A1C, percentages of saturation, and improvement in their HDL cholesterols as well their LDL cholesterol/HDL ratios.

TABLE 1:

IMPROVED LIPID PROFILES WITH WEIGHT LOSS

PT	DIET	DATE	CHOL	HDL	LDL	TG	VLDL	CHOL/HDL	WEIGHT
1	LFD	9/97	204	51	127	127	25	4.0	216
	LCD	3/98	213	73	130	80	16	3.0	202
2	LFD	5/97	264	54	171	197	N/A	4.8	N/A
	LCD	1/98	183	51	94	191	38	3.5	153
3	LFD	12/97	227	33	165	142	28	6.9	214
	LCD	3/98	248	51	169	142	28	4.8	209
4	LFD	12/97	269	56	174	153	31	4.6	185
	LCD	3/98	189	75	99	76	15	2.5	170
5	LFD	1/98	209	34	101	370	74	6.1	N/A
	LCD	4/98	187	34	116	185	37	5.5	-15
6	LFD	10/97	240	74	135	155	31	3.2	139
	LCD	3/98	295	116	138	205	41	2.5	129
7	LFD	12/97	213	62	129	115	23	3.4	N/A
	LCD	3/98	204	69	116	98	20	2.9	-12
8	LFD	10/97	170	39	87	215	43	6.7	160
	LCD	3/98	198	52	107	168	34	3.6	13
9	LFD	3/98	238	57	130	N/A	50	4.1	243
	LCD	4/98	205	64	111	155	31	3.2	194
10	LFD	1/98	191	64	115	58	78	2.9	201
	LCD	4/98	202	80	114	78	12	2.5	192
11	LFD	4/97	191	38	135	88	18	5.0	150
	LCD	3/98	237	56	163	89	18	4.2	140
12	LFD	2/98	229	38	171	102	N/A	6.0	170
	LCD	5/98	193	42	138	66	N/A	4.6	165

LFD = Low fat diet

LCD = Low carbohydrate diet

EXAMPLES:

Patient #9: Lost 30 lbs in a 4 month period Patient gained 25 lbs on a Low Fat/High Carbohydrate Diet (218 lbs up to 243 lbs) and lost 49 lbs. on the High Protein/Low Carbohydrate Plan

Patient #10: Patient weighed 201 lbs in November , 1997 started Dr. Hickey's plan and weighed 192 lbs in April 1998.

Table 2

IMPROVED HbA1C , WEIGHT LOSS & LIPID PROFILES

PT	DIET	DATE	CHOL	HDL	LDL	TG	HbA1C	CHOL/HD	WEIGHT
1	LFD	8/97	142	28	91	112	5.7	5.0	200
	LCD	3/98	186	75	86	129	5.4	2.4	170
2	LFD	12/97	178	43	126	46	7.8	4.1	N/A
	LCD	3/98	230	70	153	38	6.9	3.2	-12
3	LFD	8/97	130	32	62	172	7.8	4.0	160
	LCD	2/98	137	37	82	91	5.6	3.7	150
4	LFD	12/97	184	43	113	N/A	8.1	4.3	221
	LCD	4/98	222	71	128	N/A	5.9	3.0	205
5	LFD	12/97	299	27	239	166	6.2	11.0	186
	LCD	3/98	353	49	278	131	4.7	7.2	173
		5/98	241	37	181	117	5.5	6.5	169

HbA1C (Column 8) is the glycohemoglobin. This is the percent of saturation of the blood with sugar over the past three months. Normal non diabetic results should be less than 5.8%.

HbA1C (glycohemoglobin) above 6.4% greatly increases the complications of Diabetes Mellitis. These complications are : 1) Blindness 2) Heart attack 3) Stroke 4) Kidney Failure 5) Peripheral neuropathy and 6) Leg amputation

SUMMARY OF IMPROVED CHOLESTEROL AND BLOOD SUGAR (HbA1C) LEVELS ON A LOW CARBOHYDRATE DIET

AVERAGE WEIGHT LOSS	13 lbs.
AVERAGE IMPROVEMENT IN HDL CHOLESTEROL	47 %
AVERAGE IMPROVEMENT IN LDL CHOLESTEROL	0.8%
AVERAGE IMPROVEMENT IN VLDL CHOLESTEROL	71 %
AVERAGE TRIGLYCERIDE IMPROVEMENT	34 %
AVERAGE IMPROVEMENT IN HbA1C GLYCOHEMOGLOBIN	21 %
AVERAGE IMPROVEMENT IN TOTAL CHOLESTEROL/HDL CHOLESTEROL RATIO	43 %

GLOSSARY OF TERMS

CHOL = Total Cholesterol

HDL = High Density Lipoprotein Cholesterol (The GOOD Cholesterol)

LDL = Low Density Lipoprotein Cholesterol (The BAD Cholesterol)

VLDL = Very Low Density Lipoprotein Cholesterol (The rest of the BAD Cholesterol)

TG = Triglycerides

CHOL/HDL = The total cholesterol divided by the HDL Cholesterol ratio (you should be less than 4.0)

CHAPTER III.

THE ANATOMY OF A CLOGGED ARTERY

Insulin also promotes the blockage of arteries. What do I mean by this? The blockage of an artery is called *atherosclerosis.* The blockage or lump of junk in your vessels is called an *atheroma.* Let's take an atheroma and look at it under the microscope and discover what is there.

Atherosclerosis is an inflammatory disease. If you dissect it under the microscope you will see LDL cholesterol, which I feel is an innocent bystander, inflammatory cells called monocytes, and macrophages which are white blood cells that eat foreign material to protect us. We will find platelets which are normal cells that help us clot our blood. And we will find proteins that also help us clot blood. Some studies also show evidence of bacterial particles, thus the theory that bacteria may help create an inflammatory reaction in the blood vessel to help create a blockage.

The reason there is no firm theory on how this happens is because our state of knowledge is not yet complete on atherosclerosis. Here is the current theory. The arteries in our body have a very sophisticated internal lining called *endothelial cells.* The endothelial cell is critical to the function of the artery. It manufactures and contains chemicals that help the artery narrow or relax. These are called *prostaglandins.* The artery also contains chemicals to attract platelets and the blood clotting proteins. Certain stresses within the artery create damage in spots to the artery. High blood pressure within the artery cracks the lining or endothelial cell in spots. Sometimes this happens as an artery curves around the heart and has an increased resistance to flow. That is why with most coronary artery disease it just blocks the artery in spots and the doctors can go in with a balloon and pop that spot open so that the flow can continue. This process is called CORONARY ANGIOPLASTY or Balloon angioplasty. You may have a totally normal artery except for one single spot that clogged off. This was the site of injury to the endothelial cell that created an inflammatory reaction. This chain reaction to a clogged artery is initiated by the stress within the artery. The endothelial cell cracks and it releases a chemical that attracts platelets. Platelets are the plugs which plug the hole in the cracked artery. They are attracted to that spot immediately, as if a fire alarm went off by certain chemicals released by the endothelial cell asking for help. The platelets will then adhere to that cracked area. They in turn release other chemicals to attract the circulating protein in our body that helps us clot blood. Vitamin K is taken from leafy green vegetables and turned into proteins that help us clot our blood. These proteins will be attracted to the platelet and form a blood clot to plug the hole. If all goes well in 10 - 14 days after the lining of the blood vessel has regrown and sealed itself off, the blood clot will then be dissolved by other chemicals that are released called *plasminogen.* Tissue plasminogen is the chemical that we inject into a clogged artery to reverse a heart attack or stroke. This is a natural occurring substance in our arteries that will remove the blood clot once the endothelial cell has resealed itself and healed itself. Helping participate in this healing process is the white blood cell which generally takes away debris and aids in the inflammatory reaction.

Now, innocently enough, LDL cholesterol is coming through the artery to deliver it's cholesterol which is much needed to the cell at the end of the artery. *Free radicals*, which are created by the burning of our nutrients, are free oxygen molecules floating around in the blood with missing electrons. Oxygen is vital to our metabolism. It is used to turn food into energy. The nutrient is oxidized when it interacts with oxygen to produce energy. Remember that atoms are the basic units of all structures in nature. Atoms in turn are made up of protons positively charged at their center, and electrons negatively charged orbiting around the periphery of the atom. The number of protons and electrons differ in different chemical structures. The positive charged protons in an atom are balanced by the negative charged electrons. This is important when we refer to FREE RADICALS AND ANTIOXIDANTS.

Electrons travel in pairs. There are 3 or 4 pairs of electrons orbiting the center of an atom. When one of the pairs of electrons is broken apart in the process of oxidation during metabolism of food, that atoms energy is no longer balanced electrically. A free radical has been created. A free radical is an oxygen molecule with one electron missing from its atom. The electron was lost in the process of making energy from the nutrients in our blood. The good news is, we can take oxygen and turn food into energy by oxidation. The bad news is, this oxygen molecule is now unstable because it has donated an electron in the process. It is now electrically unstable. It is a FREE RADICAL in search of an electron to balance itself. It will attack anything to get an electron. A wrench that has been exposed to free radicals will rust after the oxidation process. A banana will turn black and ugly from free radicals attack for its electrons. Our arteries will clog and we will develop abnormal cells called cancer from free radical attack.

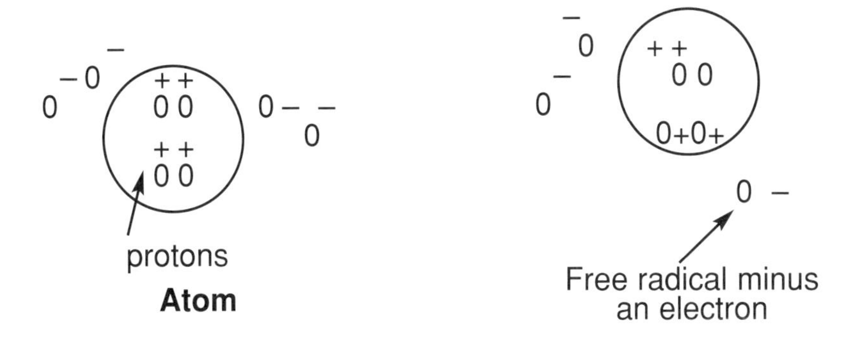

Illust. O + = Proton   O⁻ = Electron

Electrons travel in pairs....right illustration shows free radical minus electron

Free radicals are in search of electrons, so they attach themselves to a cholesterol LDL molecule. The white blood cells circulating in our blood are looking for foreigners to eat so that they can keep our body healthy. Their job is to engulf bacteria or abnormal proteins that are floating through the body. When they see this altered structure, which is not in their computer, they will eat it. When the white blood cell phagocytizes or engulfs the LDL protein, it forms what we call a FOAM cell. The foam cell looks like a white blood cell with foam inside of it's cytoplasm. This is actually the fat from the LDL cholesterol. It then goes on it's way to help in the inflammatory reaction of the blood clot and incorporates itself in the mess that is forming with the platelets and the proteins that are clogging the hole in the artery. If enough of these oxidized LDL particles get engulfed by macrophages they will form a gooey mess at that site of injury. Then, when the blood clotting needs to reverse itself, it is difficult or impossible to untangle the mess and eventually you will continue to grow more and more plaque in that spot. This mess is called *atherosclerosis* or an *atheroma*. The oxidation of LDL cholesterol can be reversed by certain vitamins called antioxidants. Vitamin E and Vitamin C, beta-carotene will be good soldiers and accept the free oxygen molecule itself, thereby destroying itself, but protecting the LDL cholesterol. In other words, the antioxidant vitamins donate their electrons to the free radicals, so that LDL Cholestrol will be left alone.

There is also a current theory that bacteria from our mouth, can get into our arteries when we go to the dentist, because he will scrub our gums. These bacteria love to intertwine with blood clot gooey substances and they in turn will promote more attraction of white blood cells. So, there is a current theory that antibiotics might some day be useful in the prevention of coronary artery disease.

There is substantial circumstantial evidence accumulating that bacteria are implicated in inflammatory reaction that leads to a ruptured plaque or atheroma. Your *coronary arteries* are the tubes that allow blood and oxygen to flow to your heart muscle. Your *carotid arteries* are the tubes or pipes leading up to your brain. They are in your neck and supply blood flow and oxygen to your brain. Your coronary and carotid arteries can be more than 90% blocked with atheroma and still not cause a heart attack or stroke. That 10% of the artery that is open may be all you need to get the oxygen to your heart or brain. However, you may get symptoms from this blocked artery.

In the case of a 90% blocked coronary artery, if your heart works too hard during exertion, your heart rate increases causing the muscle to need more oxygen than that 90% blocked artery can supply, that will make your chest pain you (angina pectoris). When you start getting chest pain, it causes you to stop what you are doing and rest. Then your heart rate slows down and the pain goes away because the reduced heart rate from resting does not require more than that 10% blood flow. You can go about your business as long as your activity does not increase your heart rate to a certain level. I have elderly patients who have over 90% blocked arteries. They only get chest pain (angina) if they walk up a certain hill or street. Because of the incline, their heart works harder and needs more oxygen. But if they avoid that hill or activity, they do not get chest pain. They have what we call *stable angina.* It is totally predictable and avoidable chest pain. My advice to them is to avoid that hill or activity and they will be fine. If they must engage in that activity, we use nitroglycerin under the tongue just before that activity. Nitroglycerin rearranges the blood flow to your heart and relaxes veins and arteries so that the work the heart must do decreases.

If your chest pain is stable or predictable, there is little fear of a heart attack. This artery is 90% blocked, but 10% open. This blockage or atheroma is usually like firm cement. It has a fibrous or hard cap on it like the cap on a tooth. You could not rupture or crack that plaque if you hit it with a hammer. If that artery slowly, completely closes off with time, it happens so gradually that other arteries usually have time to pick up the slack and reroute the blood through a detour. The blood will still get to its destination by an alternate route.

If the chest pain becomes unstable however, that means trouble. Your chest pain or severe shortness of breath (angina equivalent) was very predictable or stable until last week when it started to occur more easily with less activity and lasts a longer amount of time. Now if you walk to the bathroom you get chest pain or shortness of breath. After you eat a large meal you get the same chest pain you got when you walked up that hill. This is now called *unstable angina*. This is trouble waiting to happen .This means your artery is trying to completely close within a matter of days or even minutes. This is usually because the plaque or blockage (atheroma) has ruptured, producing the accumulation of thrombus or fresh blood clot on top of the blockage. Remember, there is no room for a blood clot in that spot, so the artery is now trying to completely close. *UNSTABLE ANGINA IS AN EMERGENCY, CALLS YOUR DOCTOR IMMEDIATELY.* If he or she tells you to take two Tylenol and call them in the morning, find another doctor. Tylenol has no anti-platelet or blood thinning properties. It is simply a pain reliever. If they tell you to take two aspirin and call them in the morning, they have reduced your chance of dying from that heart attack by about 25%. Aspirin is an anti-inflammatory drug that reduces the platelets ability to form a blood clot. That doctor at least deserves a call informing him that you have called 911 and you are on your way to the emergency room. There, your heart attack can be reversed within minutes as we will show later.

The concept of stable chest pain and unstable chest pain is important for you and your doctor to discuss. With a blood clot forming in your artery on top of a blockage, your arteries and heart do not have time to adjust. It happens too quickly. If you get chest pain after eating a meal, of course, you could have indigestion. But you better make sure that pain is not your heart warning you.

The reason we get heart pain or angina after a meal is because the artery is closing so fast that even the work of digestion is too much for it to handle. After eating, 20 - 25% of our hearts work (called cardiac output) must be pumped through your intestinal arteries to help with digestion. This is no problem unless your artery is trying to close. Getting chest pain after eating is called *postprandial angina* or after eating chest pain. It is an ominous sign and requires immediate attention.

Before getting a G.I. (gastrointestinal) series to look for indigestion or peptic ulcer, you should have your heart checked out, and by that I mean a stress test or a cardiac angiogram. Remember, that if you are in your doctors office and your chest pain is now gone, your ECG (electrocardiogram) will tell him NOTHING! Your heart is at rest and not paining you so the ECG will more than likely appear normal. Even with pain in your chest at the time of the ECG, it may appear normal at first.

I have seen many patients come into the Emergency Room with chest pain and have a normal ECG, only to have it show a heart attack 30 minutes later. The doctors index of suspicion must be high for heart disease first and foremost. After this has been ruled out with an exercise stress test or coronary angiogram, we can relax and proceed to look for other causes of chest pain. If the pain is severe or frequent, and the doctor is concerned that you are trying to close your artery, it would be more prudent to go right to the angiogram or cardiac catherization. The reason is that if the angina is unstable and the artery is trying to close, exercise on a treadmill is more dangerous than an angiogram. Angiography by the right person is very safe. This choice is based on a judgement by you and your doctor. PLEASE DO NOT BE FALSELY REASSURED BY A RESTING ECG (office or emergency room electrocardiogram).

The reason the angina becomes unstable and the chest pain occurs more easily is because the plaque in your artery has ruptured. It is provoking the formation of a blood clot (thrombus). This happens more frequently in plaque that is soft and not encapsulated by a fibrous cap. You hear about the 50 or 60 year old person who was fine in his or her doctors office today for his or her physical examination. The physical exam did not include a stress test. On the way out the door, he or she clutches their chest and drops dead. The first sign of that blocked artery was when the plaque or atheroma ruptured and the blood clot over that spot formed immediately causing sudden closure of the artery and sudden death.

The first thing the nurses in my office are trained to do in that situation is to perform CPR (cardiopulmonary resuscitation) and electrically defibrillate or shock the heart into normal rhythm. This defibrillator or electric shock devise can restart the heart, and then we can fix the artery with angioplasty by opening the artery with a balloon. If they are unable to resuscitate the patient with CPR and defibrillation, the second thing I taught them to do is to turn the patient around so that it looks like he was walking INTO my office BEFORE an exam, and not leaving after the exam.

The reason the plaque or atheroma ruptured and provoked a blood clot to form is because it became inflamed. Inflammation is what happens to your ankle when you sprain it. It becomes hot, red and swollen, due to the injury in the tissues. If your skin gets clogged, you will form a pimple, which is a combination of bacteria, white blood cells (pus), and inflammation of your skin in that area. If your underpants are too tight and they rub against your skin, that area will become inflamed and break the skin down, if you do not stop irritating it with your tight pants.

Your coronary artery atheroma or plaque also gets inflamed. It can become inflamed from friction resulting from normal blood flow past it. Inflammation of plaque can occur from free radical attack. It can occur from the toxic effects of tobacco, emotional stress (increased adrenaline), or from bacterial attack. The white blood cells in our blood release certain chemicals to help fight off tobacco toxins, bacteria, and the free radicals floating around in our blood. These chemicals may promote the rupture of plaque. Inflamed plaque is hot just like the inflammed skin when infected. Some day soon we will be able to detect the heat in your artery plaque with specialized ultra sounds of the arteries. If we could determine which plaque was hot (inflammed) and which plaque was not, we could single out those to worry about and those with stable or safe (cold) plaque.

One way researchers have recently tried to predict this is with a blood test. If you develop acute inflammation of your knee due to arthritis or gout, your knee will become hot and swollen. Your immune system will call the alarm and respond by releasing certain proteins or markers. One such protein is called C-REACTIVE PROTEIN. When one of your joints becomes inflamed, your level of c-reactive protein will start to rise in your blood because of the inflammation. If you develop high fever because of a severe infection, your body becomes inflamed and your c-reactive protein level elevates. Now we are starting to realize that when you have chest pain, or even silent coronary blockages, your c-reactive protein may predict if your artery plaque is inflamed and about to rupture. In fact, if you combined a c-reactive protein level with a total cholesterol, HDL ratio, you might be able to predict a persons first heart attack (myocardial infarction). Analysis of the Physicians Health Study involved over 14,000 apparently healthy men. They found that c-reactive protein levels total cholesterol and total cholesterol HDL ratio were each predictive of higher risk of heart attack.

Assessing both c-reactive protein and HDL cholesterol significantly improved the ability to predict heart attack risk. Compared to men whose cholesterol and c-reactive protein level were below the 75th percentile, those who had only a high total cholesterol had a relative risk of 2.3 times the normal risk of heart attack. Those who had a high c-reactive protein alone had an increased risk of 1.5 times the baseline population. But those who had high c-reactive protein levels and high cholesterol/HDL ratio had 5 times the risk of heart attack. The c-reactive protein level (a general inflammatory marker in your blood) predicated the risk of heart attack (MI) in men with both high and low cholesterol levels.[6]

This inflammation and rupture of your artery plaque may also be influenced by bacteria. Bacteria love to entwine themselves in or on uneven surfaces in our arteries and heart valves. White blood cells (monocytes, macrophages) will respond to the bacteria and release chemicals to try and kill them. These chemicals irritate the area and cause inflammation. With plaque rupture comes thrombus or blood clot. Evidence implicates Chlamydia Pneumoniae (a bacteria) and sudden rupture of atheroma in the artery. High titers of C pneumonia bacteria antibody in the blood correlates with coronary artery disease. Atherosclerotic plaques also have demonstrated these organisms within the plaque. There is some evidence that C pneumonia bacteria affects plaque stability.

The researchers of a recent study tested this theory. They wanted to see if treatment with an antibiotic to kill chlamydia would reduce:

1: unstable angina

2: heart attack

In this study, 202 patients with either of these conditions were assigned an antibiotic to kill chlamydia or placebo. The rate of unstable angina and heart attack causing death, was substantially lower in the antibiotic group, than in the placebo group.[7]

We are not completely sure what exactly causes soft silent plaque to break and cause a heart attack or stroke. It may or may not be chlamydia or some other yet unnamed bacteria or substance. But it is clear that something triggers the plague to become hot and inflamed. And all this time we thought it was just little old cholesterol. It's much more complicated than that.

It is interesting how my choice of antibiotics have changed in the last two years. Two specific bacteria we thought previously did not cause many infections in people over 50 years old are *mycoplasma and chlamydia*. The usual suspects for infections in people over 50 years old are bugs called streptococcus and hemophylus. These bacteria will be treated successfully with Penicillin based antibiotics called Cephalosporins. We have used this type of antibiotic over the years for bronchitis and sinusitis because the predominant bugs for those conditions would respond to cephalosporins. Cephalosporin antibiotics will not kill chlamydia or mycoplasma.

It is only in the last two years that studies show, that if an infection fails to respond to the usual Cephalosporin antibiotic, it may be a chlamydia or mycoplasma. A significant number with chronic bronchitis who continue to cough 6 weeks after their cephalosporin antibiotic were found to have chlamydia pneumonia. Chlamydia pneumonia will respond best or die in the presence of Tetracycline, Vibramycin, Dynabac, Zithromax and Biaxin. It was this change of antibiotic choice in the past two years that demonstrated to me the possible link between bacteria I did not previously think about and coronary artery disease in my patients.

There was an interesting case that I had in the last two years that demonstrated this point. There was a 72 year old lady who was a long term smoker, who came to my office with chest pain. Her EKG showed signs of an inferior wall ischemia, meaning she was not getting enough oxygen through the right coronary artery. I put her in the hospital, consulted a very fine cardiologist, Dr. Jamie Johnston at Hilton Head Hospital, in Hilton Head S.C. Dr. Johnston did an angiography to view the vessels and it showed that she had three arteries that were at least 90% blocked with atherosclerosis. She went for bypass surgery and did well. She had moderately severe chronic obstructive pulmonary disease from chronic cigarette smoking. She stopped smoking a few years ago, but had smoked for over 60 years. Because she had damaged her lungs significantly, she had some mild shortness of breath. But, postoperatively after her bypass surgery, she developed pneumonia. She was treated for several weeks with antibiotics and was able to get out of the hospital.

She did well for the next 2 years except for frequent bouts of acute bronchitis. This was secondary to her lung disease and her lack of defense mechanisms against bacteria. Two years after her bypass surgery she developed chest pain again. Her cholesterol was always perfect and my assumption was always that she had coronary artery disease from cigarette smoking. She had not smoked now for 5 years. She went back to Dr. Johnston, who performed another cardiac catherization and angiography. The reason for her chest pain was that at the site of insertion of one of her coronary bypass grafts, she developed a reaction and a blood clot that eventually closed off the artery. But she, to our amazement had improved the blockages in all her other arteries. The arteries that were 90% blocked had regressed and improved to 70% blockages. It was Dr. Johnston's feeling that the frequent use of antibiotics, because of her chronic bronchitis, had reduced the bacterial stimulation for developing atherosclerosis. This is not proven but a very interesting theory and it is the only way I can explain the improvement in her native arteries.

So, there is more to blocking an artery than cholesterol, and don't forget, it's the type of cholesterol that is more important than the amount of cholesterol. If you have high cholesterol and a great deal of HDL, you will actually clean out your arteries. If you have a low HDL cholesterol and a high LDL cholesterol, you will help clog your arteries.

Cholesterol is probably an innocent bystander with all the other things that go into clogging an artery. Because we have to hit a clogged artery from many aspects, it is important that we take antioxidants every day such as Vitamin E, Vitamin C, beta-carotene and selenium. They will sacrifice themselves every day to reduce the oxidized LDL and you have to replenish them every day to give yourself a new stock of antioxidants.

There is also a theory that homocystine, which is an amino acid, can provoke the scarring and inflammatory reaction in an artery. Homocysteine can stimulate the fibroblasts. The fibroblast makes scar tissue and can help harden and block arteries. We can reduce homocysteine levels by taking folic acid, 1 mg. daily. Most vitamins do not have anywhere near 1 mg. of folic acid, so you need to read the labels to see how many milligrams you are getting. Folic acid usually comes in micrograms and it takes 1000 micrograms to equal 1 mg. Studies have shown that between 1 - 5 mgs. of folic acid can reduce birth defects and coronary artery disease.

So how do we keep our arteries from clogging up? Cigarette smoke damages the endothelial cell and creates cracks. STOP SMOKING. High blood pressure puts increased force on the inside of the artery and cracks the endothelial cell setting up this inflammatory reaction to create atheroma. So we must get our blood pressure controlled to 130 for the top number and 80 for the bottom number or less. Aspirin is vital to reduce the ability of the platelet to stick or plug the crack in the endothelial cell of the artery. It is the platelet that sets off this entire reaction of blood clot and attraction of inflammatory cells. If you can reduce the platelet's ability to be attracted to the broken area, it will reduce the chance of a blockage being born. Aspirin reduces a chemical in the platelet called prostaglandins that allows the platelet to be attracted and stick to the hole in the artery. By reducing this chemical, the platelet will float on by and not cause trouble. Antioxidants such as Vitamin C, Vitamin E, beta-carotene and selenium will reduce the oxidation of LDL cholesterol and therefore reduce the chance that this taxi cab will stop at the site of vascular injury. And, finally, folic acid reduces a chemical called homocysteine, which increases the ability of the blood vessel to scar. Also, increasing HDL cholesterol will clean the cholesterol out of your arteries.

How do you improve your blood pressure, increase your HDL cholesterol, reduce your total cholesterol to HDL cholesterol ratio, and decrease oxidation of LDL cholesterol? You will do all of this if you LOSE BODY FAT. If you are getting fat eating a high carbohydrate diet, open your eyes and try something new.

Diabetic arteries block a lot differently than non-diabetic arteries. Dr. Johnston has shown me several angiograms on my diabetic patients which are distinctly different than my non-diabetic patients. When a non-diabetic patient blocks his artery, as we mentioned, it is usually just a spot or two that can be popped open with a balloon and it can be held open by the placement of a stent. A stent is a cylinder like tube or pipe that is slipped over the balloon catheter and placed in the spot where the blockage was. This prevents the blockage from rebounding and clogging the artery again. The stent is a pipe that holds the artery open and it remains there. This is the way we now treat heart attacks when they come in the emergency room. When someone is having a heart attack, we will immediately bring him to the catheterization lab at Hilton Head Hospital. Dr. Jaime Johnston or Dr. Paul Slota, interventional cardiologists, will do an immediate angiogram, find the spot that is blocked and they will pop that spot open with a balloon and slip a stent or cylinder tube over the catheter and place it at the site of that blockage so the blockage cannot collapse back down. This immediately improves blood flow to the heart and prevents muscle damage. The blockage is a combination of the atheroma or plaque that was in the vessel. This atheroma, which is now part of the lining of the blood vessel, cracks or ruptures and that attracts the platelets, protein and white blood cells to create a blood clot over that cracked area. If your artery is 60 -70% blocked at that spot by the atheroma, there is no room in the rest of the artery in that spot for a blood clot. Therefore, the artery closes off immediately and the blood flow immediately stops to that area of heart muscle.

We can also treat this with a blood thinner called TPA (tissue plasminogen activator). This is the natural occurring blood thinner that takes the clot away during natural anticoagulation. But, because we don't have time to wait for that process to happen, we can inject TPA into the vein and it will dissolve that clot. It will not get rid of the atheroma, but it will at least open up the artery enough to save the heart. A better way of doing this is to directly open the artery with angioplasty and stent placement.

CORONARY ARTERIES

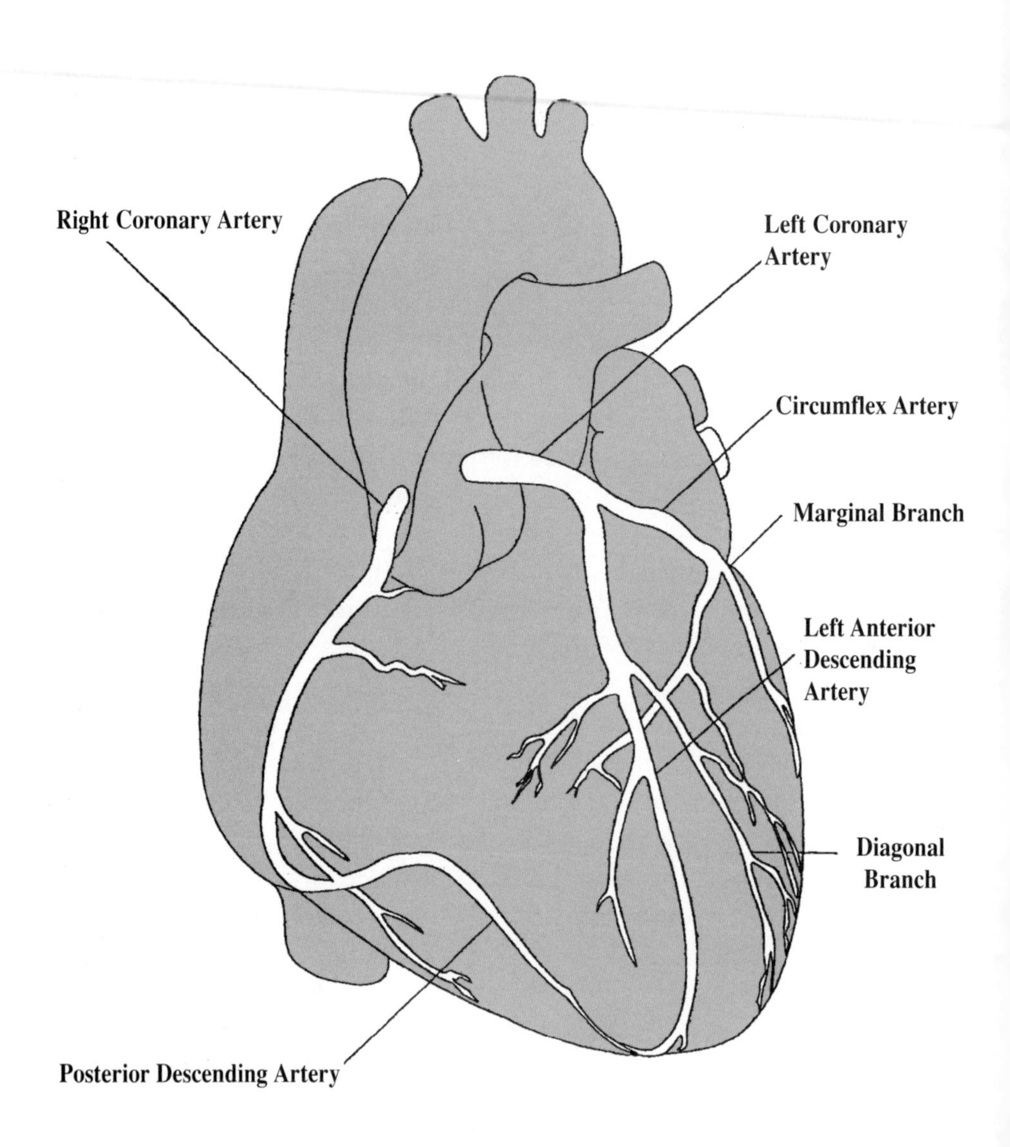

The Normal Artery and its Inhabitants
Normal Blood Pressure 120/80

I

ARTERY

SMOOTH MUSCLE

ENDOTHELIAL CELL LINING

Platelets

LDL - Cholesterol

Clotting Proteins

O_2 (Oxygen)

White Blood Cell

ENDOTHELIAL CELL LINING

SMOOTH MUSCLE

II

THE BIRTH OF AN ATHEROMA OR BLOCKAGE
It starts with a crack in the endothelial lining.
The platelets, clotting proteins and white blood cells try to help by plugging the hole or crack

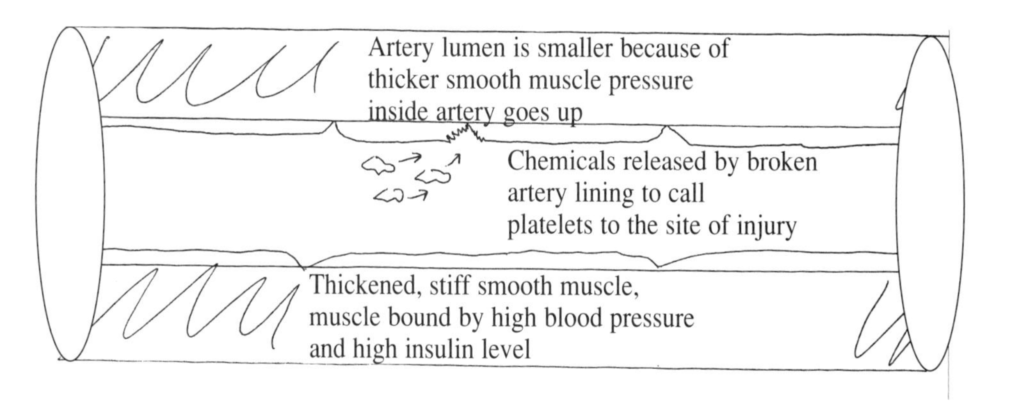

III

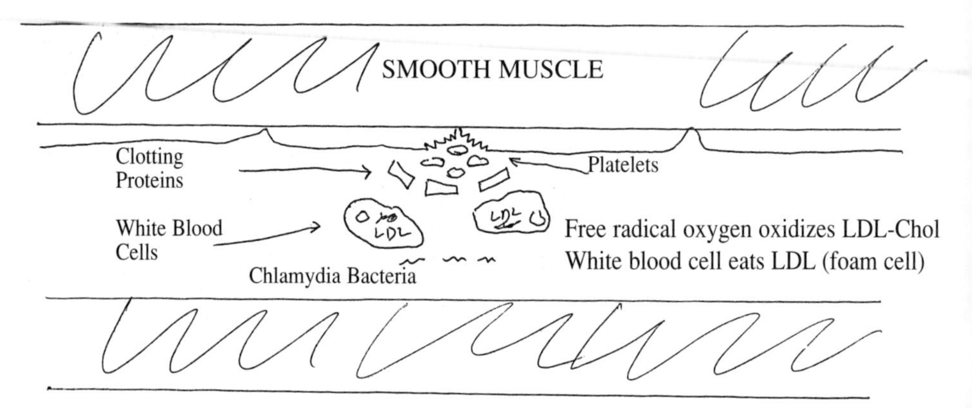
ARTERY
SMOOTH MUSCLE
Clotting Proteins
Platelets
White Blood Cells
LDL
LDL
Free radical oxygen oxidizes LDL-Chol
White blood cell eats LDL (foam cell)
Chlamydia Bacteria

IV

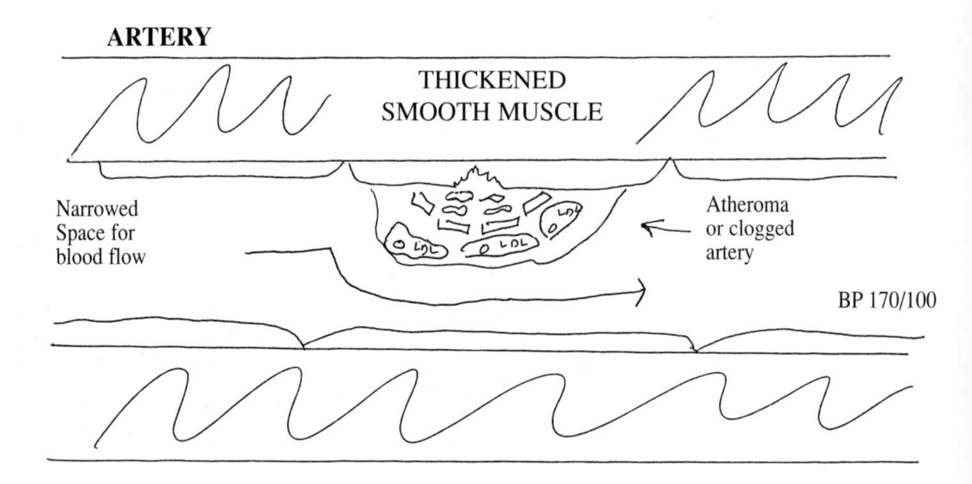
ARTERY
THICKENED SMOOTH MUSCLE
Narrowed Space for blood flow
LDL
LDL
Atheroma or clogged artery
BP 170/100

The Anatomy of a Heart Attack or Thrombotic Stroke

I

ARTERY

THICKENED
SMOOTH MUSCLE
Platelets
HELP
Plaque Ruptures
or Fractures
due to force within
the artery

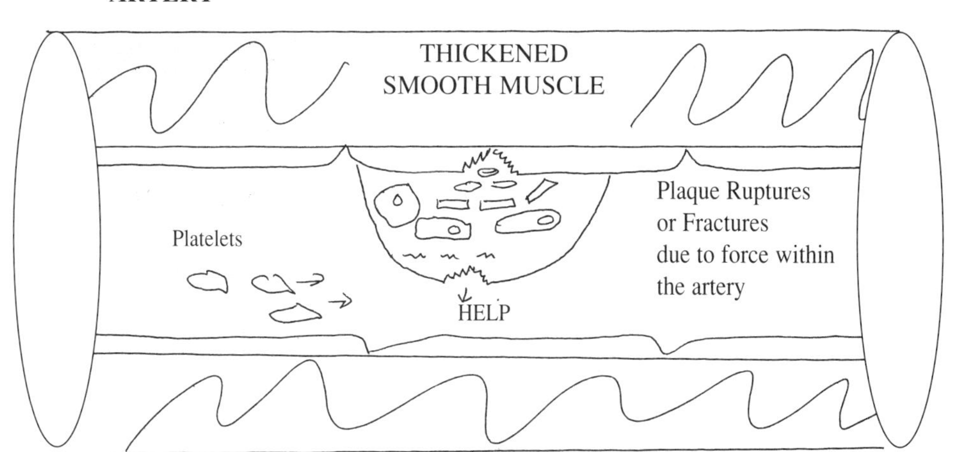

II

ARTERY

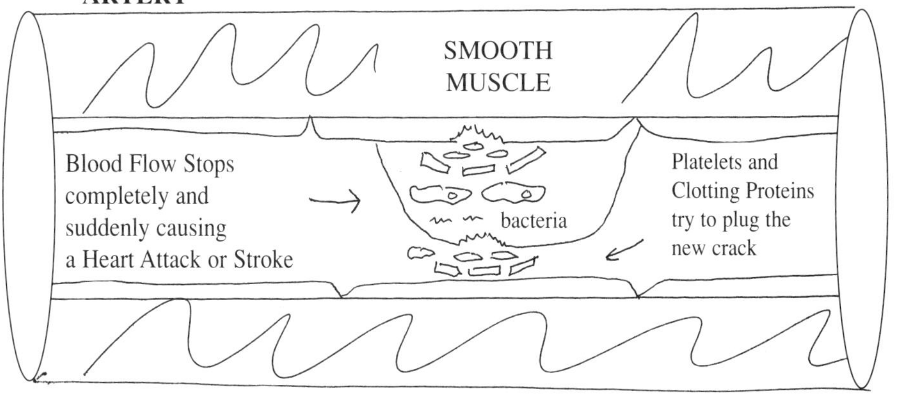

SMOOTH
MUSCLE
Blood Flow Stops
completely and
suddenly causing
a Heart Attack or Stroke
bacteria
Platelets and
Clotting Proteins
try to plug the
new crack

Complete and Sudden Blockage of the Artery

I

THE DOCTOR TO THE RESCUE

Clot Buster Injection
Tissue Plasminogen Activator
or Streptokinase injection

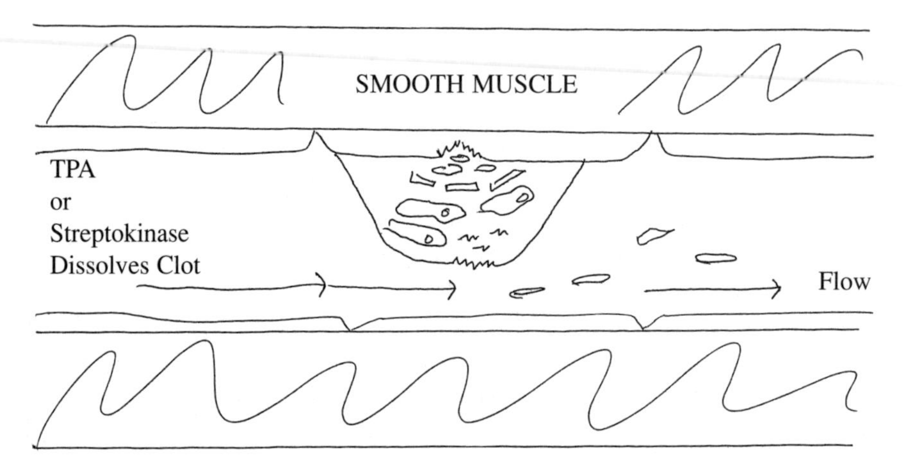

Plaque remains, but clot (thrombus) is dissolved.
Blood flow is restored to the Heart or Brain
in minutes after injection.
This will open 65 percent of thrombosed
(blood clot) arteries.

BALLOON ANGIOPLASTY AND STENT PLACEMENT FOR AN ACUTELY BLOCKED ARTERY

The catheter is placed in the groin (femoral artery) and pushed up to the heart arteries (coronaries) through the aorta

I

ARTERY

SMOOTH MUSCLE

Plaque

Balloon Catheter

Thrombus or clot

II

ARTERY

SMOOTH MUSCLE

Balloon Catheter placed through the Atheroma and Clot

III

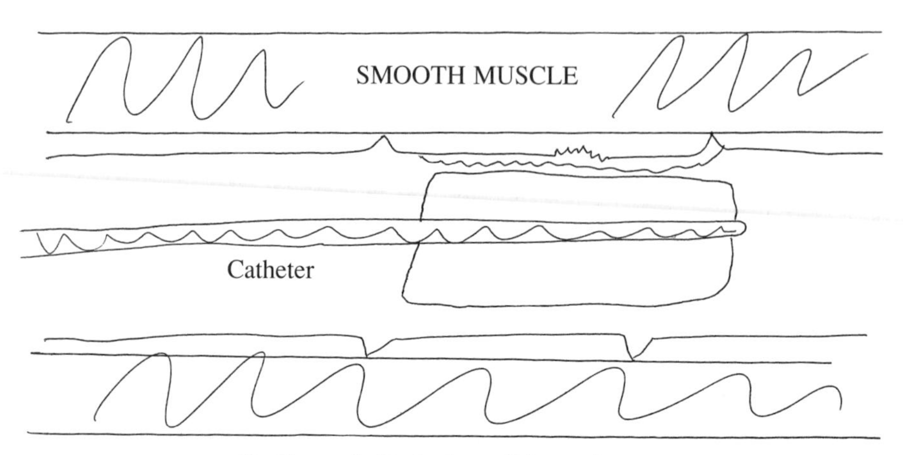

Balloon inflated pushing plaque and thrombus aside

IV

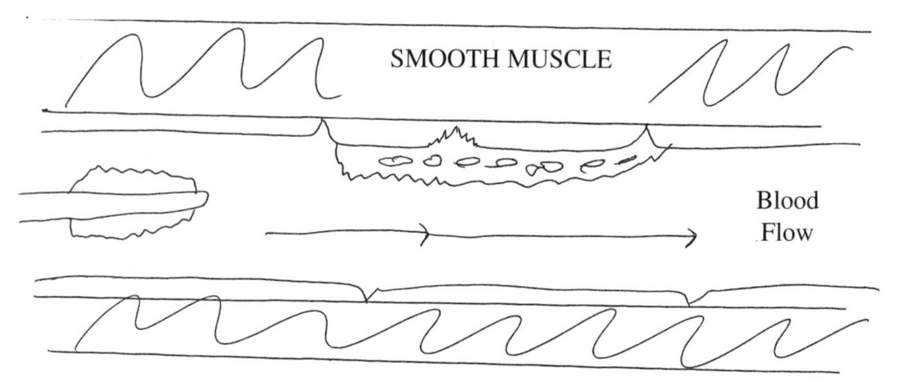

Balloon deflated after successful angioplasty plaque and clot reduced. Artery now open heart gets relief.

V

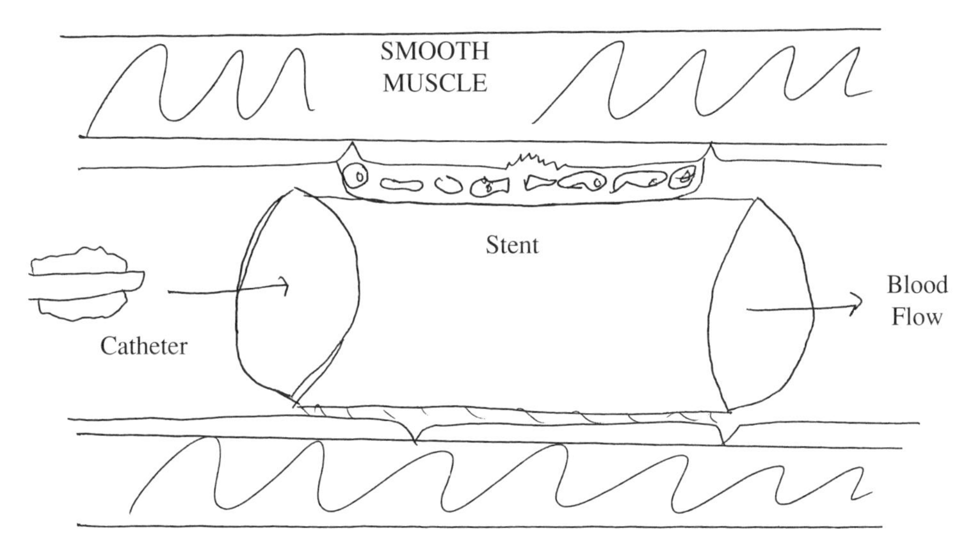

Stent is slipped over the Balloon Catheter and secures the artery in that spot. It remains in the artery at that spot permanently, preventing the plaque from collapsing back down and occluding the artery again. Balloon angioplasty and stent placement is 99 percent effective in restoring blood flow and reversing a heart attack.

OUNCE OF PREVENTION

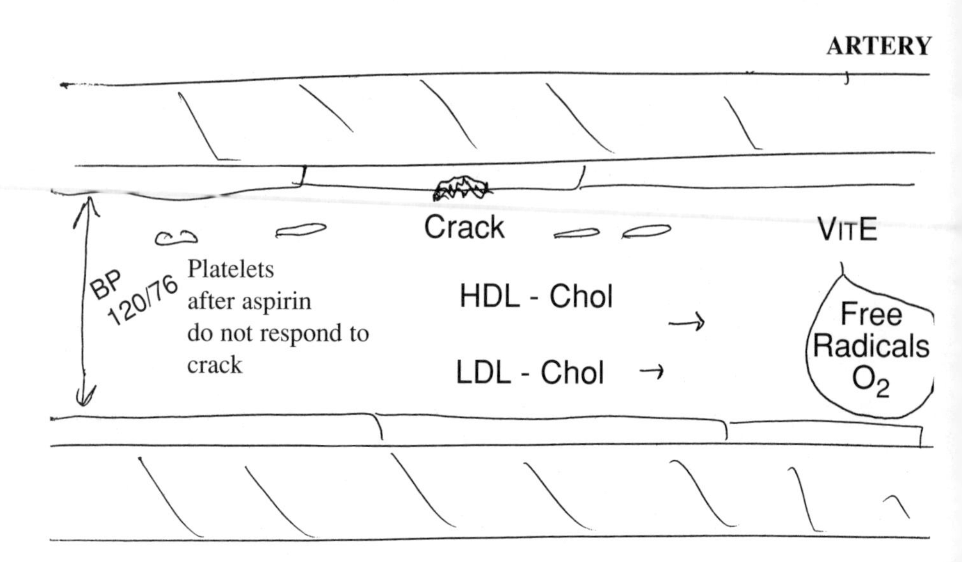

PREVENTION OF ATHEROSCLEROSIS

1. Aspirin reduces platelets tendency to plug the small cracks in the arteries. The platelets start the whole ball rolling toward an atheroma. The small cracks will heal by themselves if left alone.

2. Increase HDL cholesterol. It will not stick to the artery wall.

3. Antioxidants prevent oxygen free radicals from oxidizing LDL - cholesterol. LDL then does not stop at site of injury.

4. Reducing Hyperinsulin in blood vessel, reduces blood pressure and muscle stiffness. The artery is then more relaxed and the internal pressure is reduced. This reduces the cracks in the endothelial lining.

5. Folic acid reduces the scar tissue that develops after the lining is injured.

Unfortunately, Balloon Angioplasty is usually not possible in the diabetic. The diabetic artery blocks in a different manner than the non diabetic artery. The reason for this difference is increased sugar levels that circulate through the arteries and the consequence of that increased insulin levels. Insulin increases smooth muscle hypertrophy. Smooth muscle is an important part of the artery to allow the artery to relax and contract. When you are running around the track and it is 90 degrees, you will increase your body heat and you will need to get rid of that heat circulating your blood to the skin. The arteries will relax and open and the blood will flow to your skin carrying the heat which will be evaporated from your body with sweat. In the process, the increased blood flow creates increased heat and redness to your skin so you become flushed. On the contrary, when it is cold, your body wants to conserve heat so you will constrict the arteries flowing into your extremities and into your skin and reduce the blood flow, that is why you get pale or blue when you are frigid and your skin will be cold. The arteries in the skin as well as the arteries in the heart require this ability to relax and to constrict. The smooth muscles within the artery allows this to happen. Carbohydrates or sugars stimulate insulin at increased levels in your blood. Insulin creates hypertrophy or enlargement of the muscles inside the arteries and this creates a more narrow artery. It is interesting that Dr. Johnston and Dr. Slota have often commented to me that diabetic arteries are smaller than non diabetic.

Well, actually they have grown smaller because of insulin stimulation to the smooth muscle. This increases friction and pressure within the artery and increases the likelihood that the artery will break down in several spots. When you look at a diabetic's artery who is having chest pain, they usually have what we call DIFFUSE DISEASE. The entire artery looks diseased and it is very difficult to do angioplasty on their arteries. Their arteries are more fragile and there is not just one spot, but several different spots that are clogged or blocked. So it is not a matter of going in with a balloon and popping open the one bad spot. You have to bypass the entire vessel with a new artery. So, often times, diabetics require bypass surgery because they have their entire artery involved in atherosclerosis. Insulin is <u>their</u> problem. Insulin is <u>our</u> problem. Reduce circulating insulin levels and you will be healthier. This increased insulin stimulation of the smooth muscle of the artery which occurs in obese people, as well as in diabetics, increases the size of the muscle to the artery, making it more narrow.

This is a contributing factor to developing high blood pressure. Since that artery is more narrow, but the heart is still pumping with the same force, the pressure has to go up in the artery. This insulin stimulation by carbohydrates can create high blood pressure simply by making your arteries smaller and less flexible. I know I'm going against the *GRAIN*, with all due respect to my colleagues, but they're wrong. INSULIN and CARBOHYDRATES are the enemy, not cholesterol.

CHAPTER IV.

THE INSULIN REGULATING, LOW CARBOHYDRATE DIET

Now we will come to the part of the book that will help you learn how to use foods to your advantage and to take advantage of your internal hormones. First of all, we need to discuss the sugar content of foods. This concept is called the GLYCEMIC INDEX or how much insulin is induced by that food. Obviously, a food that induces a very rapid and high blood sugar within an hour of eating, will induce a high circulating insulin level that will cause all of the problems that I have been discussing. Some doctors from Canada, Jenkins, et al., decided to test the sugar response from foods. They tested foods against pure sugar or glucose. They placed several teaspoons of sugar (100 grams of glucose) in a glass of water and had people drink the sugar water and then measured how HIGH the sugar level went and how FAST it went up in the blood. They also measured how much insulin was induced by that rapid sugar rise in the blood. They then compared other foods to this. They called the glycemic effect of pure sugar and water 100%. They tested foods against this to see whether it would be above pure sugar's ability to raise sugar or below pure sugar's ability to raise your total blood sugar. If you eat foods that have a glycemic index of less than 30, you will get a very small rise in sugar and consequently a very small amount of insulin in your blood. If you have a small amount of insulin after a meal, you will not get fat. If you have a large amount of insulin after a meal you will increase fat storage and fat production. That is why carbohydrates before exercise are ridiculous. They will prevent you from losing fat. They will give you energy, but they will not do what most of us exercise for, that is the loss of body fat. Plain water is the best thing to drink before exercise.

It is interesting to see that some foods actually raise your blood sugar higher and faster than pure sugar. Examples are corn flakes, puffed wheat, french bread, instant white rice, 40% bran flakes, rice krispies and rice cakes. I often ate rice cakes because they had no fat content and I thought they were a good healthy snack to help me lose weight. I now see that they have a glycemic index greater than 100%. They have the ability to raise my blood sugar and insulin levels faster and higher than pure sugar. Foods with a glycemic index equal to pure sugar are white bread and whole wheat bread. Foods with a glycemic index between 90 and 99%, which is close to pure sugar, are Grape-nuts cereal, carrots, shredded wheat, corn chips and apricots. I bet you never thought that carrots could make you fat. Foods with a glycemic index of between 80 and 89% are white rice, white potatoes, corn, rye bread, bananas, mangos and papaya. Foods with a low glycemic index, between 40 and 49% are sweet potatoes, grapes, oranges, and whole grain rye bread. The glycemic index between 30 and 39% include such foods as apples, pears, tomato soup, ice cream (interestingly enough), milk and yogurt. The lowest glycemic index of foods with carbohydrates in them are lentils, plums, peaches, grapefruits, cherries, soybean and peanuts. Actually, the fat in peanuts slows down the carbohydrate absorption. If a carbohydrate substance has fat in it, it buffers and reduces the flow of sugar into the blood so it flows more slowly. That is why peanuts and walnuts as well as almonds are good snack foods. I will list for you as thoroughly as possible all the foods that were tested and their glycemic index at the end of the book in the reference table section. Remember though, whether it is a low glycemic index or a high glycemic index, it is still carbohydrates. Obviously, if one has to get some variety in his diet, you should tend more towards the lower glycemic index and stay under 30 - 39% glycemic index.

Foods that rank lower on the index list help maintain your weight, balance your sugar and give you more energy. Eating protein and fat with your lower glycemic foods will buffer the flow of carbohydrates into the blood and slow down the insulin response.

Foods with a zero glycemic index are eggs, meat, poultry, cheese, mayonnaise , shellfish, fish and all the things you were told not to eat for the past 20 years. These will not stimulate insulin and you will lose weight if you eat them. To make this diet work, especially initially, it is important to reduce your carbohydrate intake to less than *30 GRAMS A DAY*. A slice of bread has 15 grams of carbohydrates, a banana has 20 grams of carbohydrates .

PREFERRED BREAKFAST FOODS

Eggs are the healthiest food we have. I think you should rely upon eggs as much as possible. I am not afraid of egg yolk because I am not afraid of cholesterol. Remember, if it is good cholesterol or HDL cholesterol that is flowing around, it actually protects you. You will only stimulate bad (LDL or VLDL) cholesterol by carbohydrate and insulin stimulation. So, don't be afraid to eat eggs. They should be your staple.

If you have to have breakfast cereal, you must find one with very high fiber content such as Fiber One. The reason for this is that fiber is not digestible by the human intestines. When you see fiber grams in a substance, you know that it is not going to contribute any nutrition to the body. It will provide bulk to the intestine and will actually reduce the absorption of other carbohydrates. So fiber is a very positive thing. If you must have breakfast cereal, find one with a very high fiber content. But I recommend sticking with eggs at first. I would have fried or soft boiled eggs with bacon, Canadian bacon, or sausage. No toast, please, until our weight loss is accomplished. Toast, again , has a glycemic index of 100% similar to pure sugar. It will raise your insulin level and you will store everything you eat. If you don't eat toast, you can have all the bacon and eggs you want and they will be burned up as energy and not stored as fat. You can have cheese omelettes with peppers and onions. If you must have oatmeal, it must be the slow cooking variety that simmers overnight. The instant varieties have very high sugar contents and very high glycemic indexes. So rely upon eggs and bacon and sausage for breakfast.

Fruit juices are not a good idea, again, because they are concentrated carbohydrates and will raise your blood sugar. If you must have fruit juices, you must drink them at least an hour before or two hours after your meal. This is the way you should eat fruit also. Fruit should be eaten by itself. Fruit have very few carbohydrates in the form of fructose, so that they have a low glycemic index. The exception to this are bananas and raisins, which should be avoided. But, even the low glycemic index of fruit will stimulate insulin and if you have other food in your blood, they will be stored rather than used as energy. So, eat your fruit by itself, alone as a snack. Make sure it is not around your meals. That is why you should avoid fruit juice with your breakfast. Obviously, any type of meat or eggs is okay for breakfast. There are no carbohydrates at all in that breakfast.

PREFERRED LUNCH FOODS

Foods to avoid are breakfast cereals, fruit juices, bagels, toast, waffles and pancakes. All with a very high carbohydrate content. Your mid morning snack can be a piece of fruit or some cheese. Remember to take it at least two hours after you have eaten your breakfast.

For lunch I would prefer that you stick with tuna salad with real mayonnaise, chicken salad or egg salad. You can also have lettuce and cucumbers. Remember, you don't have to count your calories so you can have a significant bowl of tuna or chicken salad. But, PLEASE, no bread. Mayonnaise is fine since it is a monounsaturated fat which actually lowers cholesterol and improves HDL cholesterol. I don't want to use any LOW FAT mayonnaise or mixers, because if it is low fat, it almost always means high sugar. You can have meat and cheese for lunch, but no bread. That means cold cuts, cheese, chicken, turkey or fish. Shellfish and shrimp are also fine, but be careful of the cocktail sauce which may have a high carbohydrate content. I would prefer that you use butter or some low carbohydrate flavored cocktail mix.

PREFERRED DINNER FOODS

For dinner, you can have any type of meat including pork, lamb, beef, chicken, turkey, steak, sausage, lobster, shellfish, clams, regular fish of any type. However, be very careful not to bread these in bread crumbs or any types of batter which is high in carbohydrates. If you still don't believe my theory on fat not being harmful, you can obviously trim the fat off of beef, take the skin off of chicken and reduce your saturated fat. It will still work as long as you don't take carbohydrates.

If you want to lose weight, especially in the first three months, you must avoid bread, rice, pasta, potatoes, corn, carrots, beets, peas, cookies, cake and candy. Avoid them and you will lose substantial amounts of weight. You should keep your carbohydrate grams below 30 grams a day for the first month. If you find you are not losing enough weight, cut it down to 20 grams a day. In three months, you should see at least 15 or 20 pounds of weight loss. If you want to continue to lose weight, continue to keep your carbohydrate intake between 20 and 30 grams. If necessary, drop it below 20 grams.

As you get towards your ideal weight, the weight that you are happy and satisfied with, and you see improvement in your cholesterol, blood pressure and blood parameters, you may start to increase your carbohydrate intake. Remember, this is what got you fat in the first place. NEVER FORGET IT! But you probably can increase your intake gradually, to see what level it takes to make you fat. It could be 50 grams, 80 grams or 100 grams of carbohydrate. That is individual for each person. The first carbohydrates I would introduce, with the exception of banana and raisins, are fruits. Fruit is healthy and has a low carbohydrate glycemic index. It is also sweet and satisfies the sweet tooth. I would be very cautious with bread, rice and pasta and also cautious with white potatoes. But you can enjoy these once your weight is down to where you want it to be. Just remember, they should be OCCASIONAL, and not part of your steady diet. We feed our cattle and pigs, grains and corn to make them fat. It stands to reason, they will make us fat for slaughter also. So stay away from the big five: bread, rice , pasta, potatoes and corn. Beware of the carbohydrate intake of foods. Many of my patient's eat anything they want after they achieve their weight loss. But they are careful once their weight starts climbing up, to restrict the carbohydrates and go back to what got them feeling well. This kind of variety makes it pleasant, and remember, there is no calorie counting. You don't need to count calories. Just count carbohydrate grams. So restrict your carbohydrates to less than 30 grams and decrease further, if your weight loss does not occur. Restrict it to less than 20 grams if necessary. I will provide for you a thorough listing of the carbohydrate grams of all foods. You may feel negative about this since it is going against the GRAIN, and I understand that. I felt negative about it also because of my background and my study as a physician. The only reason I turned to this is because nothing I was doing was working. I followed all the rules for so many years and my patient's were not benefitting. I had the fortitude to do something different because my true interest was improvement in the blood pressure, cholesterol, blood sugar and body weight of my patients. I am as shocked as you are that this works, but it does.

I think the bottom line is, does it work for you? Certainly eating this way is not going to cause you any harm for three to four months. Atherosclerosis or atheromas take many years, probably 30 years to develop. What I would do is your own scientific experiment. If you do this for three months and you feel better, your cholesterol and body weight are better, as measured by your doctor, then you have helped yourself. You will be the best judge of that. You will know if you feel better, if you have more energy and you will see the results in your HDL cholesterol. Certainly, if you are diabetic, you will see the ability to control your sugar without medications. If it doesn't help you, obviously, don't do it. But my reason for turning to this type of diet was because the low fat, high complex carbohydrate diet I've followed for years, was a miserable failure.

This diet is not difficult. Especially, if you follow it STRICTLY for the first three months. Eat anything that does not have a great deal of carbohydrates in it and learn to COUNT YOUR CARBOHYDRATES. Rely on the listing of foods that shows the carbohydrate grams and try and count them as best as you can.

There are certain vitamins and minerals that are essential to help your metabolism burn fat and to protect you arteries from atherosclerosis. The next chapter will discuss these vitamins and the ones that I feel are essential to help you to a thinner and more healthy, energetic, lifestyle.

GUIDELINES FOR HICKEY DIET PROGRAM

Key Component for Weight Loss:

1. Must get sugar/carbohydrates out of Diet !!
2. Carbohydrates cause insulin to be released into system, in turn insulin enhances the burning of sugar while inhibiting the burning of fats. Not a good combination when trying to lose Fat!
3. Reduce the secretion of insulin into the system by taking in primarily Protein and Fats.
4. Keep carbohydrate intake to 20 grams or less until half of ideal bodyweight is reached.

Recommended Lists of Foods:

1. Any kind of meat (steak, beef, chicken, pork, bacon etc.)
2. Eggs
3. Some vegetables
    - a.)Unlimited salad with real dressing
    - b.) Green beans
    - c.) Asparagus
    - d.) Broccoli/squash/zucchini
    - e.) Dark green and/or yellow vegetables
4. Sugar free Jell-O with real whipped cream
5. Wheat bran cereal (small amount) , Shredded wheat (small amount)
6. Red Wine or Dry White Wine (6oz has3.0 carbohydrates), or Light Beer
7. Fruit if eaten 1/2 hour before a meal or 2 hours after a meal (this fruit must count into your carbohydrate count !!)
8. Real cheese, not fat-free.
9. Recommended vitamins: a multivitamin, 600 mcg of chromium polynicotinate, folic acid (which may be in the multivitamin) and an antioxidant with B complex

Avoid List of Foods:

1. Bread, Rice , Pasta, Potatoes
2. Corn
3. Beets
4. Sweets, cookies, cake (even fat~free)
5. Breakfast cereals
6. Carrots
7. Black beans, navy beans, peas, etc.
8. Anything with carbohydrates!!!!

For breakfast you could have bacon and eggs (NO Toast) or a Cheese Omelet. For lunch you can have Egg Salad, Chicken Salad, Tuna Salad, etc. with REAL mayo. Or perhaps a Grilled Chicken Salad with Real Ranch, Bleu Cheese or Caesar dressing. For dinner you could have a steak with a tossed salad and green beans. For dessert you can have sugar free Jell-o with a little real whipped cream. Snack on beef jerky, nuts, cheese (REAL) or celery.

Carbohydrate Gram List

Alcohol and Mixers

Food	Amount	Carbohydrate Gram
Beer		
Becks	12 oz	10.0
Bud Lite	12 oz.	6.9
Budweiser	12 oz.	11.3
Busch	12 oz.	11.9
Coors	12 oz.	11.6
Coors Lite	12 oz.	5.0
KeyStone(Dry)	12 oz.	6.4
KeyStone(Light)	12 oz.	4.4
Killians	12 oz.	15.0
Michelob Light	12 oz.	11.9
Miller	12 oz.	13.1
Miller Lite	12 oz.	3.2
Zima	12 oz.	14.0
Bloody Mary	8 oz.	7.8
Club Soda	8 oz.	0.0
Daiquiri	8 oz.	16.4
Fuzzy Naval	8 oz.	42.6
Ginger Ale	1 C.	20.8
Lime Juice	1/4 C.	5.5
Liquor	1 oz.	0.0
(Bourbon/Gin/Rum/Vodka)		
Long island ice tea	8oz.	16.9
Manhattan	8 oz.	7.2
Martini	8 oz.	0.7
Non-alcoholic beer	12 oz.	5.0
Perrier	8 oz.	0.0
Pina colada	8 oz.	72.0
Rum carbonated	8 oz.	18.4
Scotch and Soda	8 oz.	0.1
Tom collins	8 oz.	3.0
Tonic	8 oz.	20.8
Vermouth (dry)	1 item	1.0
(sweet)	1 item	12.0
White Russian	8oz.	38.4

Food		Amount	Carbohydrate Gram
Wine	(Red)	4 oz.	2.0
	(White)	4 oz.	2.0

Bean

Food	Amount	Carbohydrate Gram
Baked	1/2 C.	26.0
Bean Dip	1 T.	2.5
Black eyed peas	1/2 C.	15.0
Black	1/2 C.	17.0
Green Bean	1/2 C.	4.3
Cow Peas	1/2 C.	8.5
Kidney	1/2 C.	20.0
Lima	1/2 C.	63.5
Navy	1/2 C.	64.0
Peas green	1/2 C.	13.5
Pinto	1/2 C.	61.0
Refried	1/2 C.	20.0
Wax	1/2 C.	4.0
White (great northern)	1/2 C.	18.6

Beverages

Food		Amount	Carbohydrate Gram
Crystal Light		8 oz.	0.0
Lemonade		1 C.	26.0
Milk	(Whole)	1 C.	11.4
	(1%)	1 C.	11.7
	(2%)	1 C.	11.7
	(Skim)	1 C	11.9
	(Chocolate)	1 C.	25.0
Soft Drinks	(Coke)	8 oz.	28.9
	(Diet Coke)	8 oz.	0.1
Tea		8 oz.	0.7
Herbal Tea		8 oz.	0.5

Cereal

Food	Amount	Carbohydrate Gram
AllBran	1 C.	44.0
Kellogg's Bran Complete	1 C.	33.3
Cheerios	1 C.	23.0
Cornflakes	1 C.	26.0
Crispix	1 C.	27.0
FiberOne	1 C.	48.0
Frosted Mini Wheats	1 C.	45.0
Frosted Flakes	1 C.	37.0
Grapenuts	1 C.	91.0
Oatmeal (cooked)	1 C.	25.0
Puffed Rice	1 C.	12.0
PuffedWheat	1 C.	9.4
Raisin Bran	1 C.	43.0
Special K	1 C	21.0

Cheese

Food	Amount	Carbohydrate Gram
American	1 oz.	2.0
Blue	1 oz	0.6
Cheddar	1 oz.	0.5
Cheese Food Kraft Slices	1 oz.	2.5
Cheese Food Jalepeno Kraft	1 oz.	2.7
Cheese Whiz & Hot Salsa	1 T.	1.0
Cottage (1%)	1 C.	6.1
(2%)	1 C.	8.2
Feta	1 oz.	1.1
Gouda	1oz.	0.6
Limburger	1 oz.	0.1
Monterey Jack	1 oz.	0.2
Muenster	1 slice	0.5
Mozzarella	1 oz.	0.8
Parmesan	1 oz.	0.2
Philadelphia Cream Cheese	1 T.	1.0
Provolone	1 oz.	0.2
Ricotta	1 C.	7.4
Roquefort	1 oz.	0.5

Dessert

Food		Amount	Carbohydrate Gram
Blueberry muffin		1 each	27.0
Bran muffin		1 each	19.0
Brownie Double Fudge		1 each	29.0
Chocolate cake w/o icing		1 slice	30.0
Chocolate chip cookie		1 each	9.1
Chocolatesandwichcookie		1 each	7.0
Cookie (plain)		1 each	7.7
Donut (glazed)		1 each	25.0
English muffin		1 each	26.0
Fig bar		1 each	11.0
Pudding	(SFChoc. Jello)	1/2 C.	7.0
	(SF Vanilla)	1/2 C.	5.0
	(Choc)	1/2 C	22.0
	(Lemon)	1/2 C.	24.0
	(Rice)	1/2 C	40.0
Sugar cookie		1 each	10.2
Jello (sugar~free)		1 C.	0.0

Dishes

Food	Amount	Carbohydrate Gram
Bean Burrito (TacoBell)	1 each	54.0
Beef stew	1 C.	15.0
Chicken ala king	1 C.	9.9
Chicken cacciatore	1 C.	5.2
Chicken cordon bleu	3.5 oz.	4.1
Chicken fajitas (w/shell)	8 oz.	20.0
Chicken parmesan	7 oz.	22.4
Chicken parmigiana	1 serving (11.5 oz.)	47.0
Chow mein	1 C.	18.0
Manicotti	1 serving	32.0
Pizza	1 slice	19.0
Ravioli	4 oz.	28.0
Tamale	6.8 oz	23.0

Fruit List

Food	Amount	Carbohydrate Gram
Apple (2 1/4 inch diameter)	1/2	10.5
Banana	1/2	13.0
Apricot (no pk)	1/2	8.0
Applesauce (can unsweetened)	1/2	13.8
Blackberry (Frzn unsweetened)	1/2 C.	12.0
Raw	1/2 C.	9.0
Blueberry (raw)	1/2 C.	10.2
Cantaloupe (raw cubed)	1/2 C.	6.6
Cherries (sour red)	1/2 C.	9.4
(red maraschino)	1 each	3.0
(sour canned water pk.)	1/2 C	10.5
(sour red canned light)	1/2 C.	24.0
Cranberry (raw)	1/2 C.	58.5
Fig (raw)	1 each	9.0
Grapefruit (raw)	1/2 C.	9.2
Grapes	1/2 C.	7.8
Guava (raw)	1/2 C.	5.3
Honey Dew (raw cubed)	1/2 C.	7.8
Kiwi (raw)	1/2 C.	5.5
Lemon (raw)	1 each	5.4
Lime (raw)	1 each	7.6
Mango (raw)	1/2 item	17.6
Nectarine (raw)	1 item	16.0
Orange (raw)	1/2 C.	7.7
Papaya (raw)	1/2 C.	6.8
Passion fruit (raw)	1 item	0.6
Peach (raw)	1/2 item	48
Peach (water packed)	1/2 C	7.0
Pineapple (raw)	1/2 C.	9.6
Plum (raw)	1 each	6.0
Prune (dried w/o sugar)	1/2 C.	30.0
(raw)	1 each	6.0
(stewed)	1 each	6.0
(heavy syrup)	1/2 C.	32.0
Raisin (seedless)	1/2 C	62.0
Raspberry (raw)	1/2 C.	7.1

Food	Amount	Carbohydrate Gram
Strawberry (raw)	1/2 C	5.0
Tangerine (raw)	1/2 C.	4.7
Watermelon (raw cubed)	1/2 C.	5.7

Fruit Juice

Food	Amount	Carbohydrate Gram
Apple Cider	1/2 C.	17.1
Apple Juice	1/2 C.	14.5
Cranberry Cocktail	1/2 C.	18.2
Cranberry Juice	1/2 C.	18.3
Grape Juice	1/2 C.	11.1
Grapefruit Juice	1/2 C.	11.1
Lemon Juice	1/2 C.	10.5
Orange Juice	1/2 C.	12.3
Prune Juice	1/2 C.	22.0

Ice Cream

Food	Amount	Carbohydrate Gram
Vanilla	1 C.	19.0
Butter Pecan	1 C.	44.0
Cheesecake (Edys)	1 C.	32.0
Chocolate	1 C.	37.0
No Sugar Added (Edys)	1 C.	26.0
Peach Sorbet	1 C.	20.0
Pistachio	1 C.	34.0
Sorbet	1 C.	34.0
Sorbet (Baskin and Robbins)	1 C.	60.0
Sorbet (low calorie w/aspartame)	1 C	3.2
Sherbet	1 C.	58.0
Ice cream cone (no ice cream)	1 each	84
Ice cream bar (cappuccino blast)	1 each	18.0
Haagen Daz Almond	1 each	25.0

Meat

Food	Amount	Carbohydrate Gram
Abalone (steamed or poach)	1 oz.	3.3
Bacon	1 slice	.1
Beef (ground)	3 oz.	0.0
(dried)	1 slice	0.1
Braunschweiger	1 slice	0.5
Canadian bacon	1 slice	.4
Capon	1 each	0.0
Chicken	1 pc.	0.0
Chicken salad (commercial)	1 C.	17.4
Corned beef	1 oz.	0.0
Cornish hen	1 each	0.0
Crab	1 each	0.0
(imitation)	3 oz.	8.6
Duck	3 oz.	0.2
Egg (chicken)	1 each	0.6
Flounder	3 oz.	0.4
Frankfurter	1 item	1.4
Grouper	3 oz.	0.0
Haddock	3 oz.	0.0
Halibut	3 oz.	0.0
Ham	3 oz.	0.0
Ham salad	1 C.	25.6
Kielbasa (beef or pork)	1 slice	0.5
Lamb	3 oz.	0.0
Liver	3 oz.	4.8
Lunch meat		
Liverwurst	1 slice	0.4
bologna	1 slice	0.7
ham	1 C.	0.0
Healthy Choice ham	1 slice	0.3
Healthy Choice turkey/ Roast beef	1 slice	0.3
Mussel	1 oz.	3.3
Oyster	1 oz.	1.5
Pork	3 oz.	0.0
Rabbit	3 oz.	0.0

Food	Amount	Carbohydrate Gram
Ribs	3 oz.	0.0
Salmon	3 oz.	0.0
Sardine	1 oz.	0.0
Sausage (Italian)	1 item (2.6oz.)	1.0
(Bratwurst/smoked)	3 oz.	1.5
Swordfish	3 oz.	0.0
Tofu (firm)	3 oz.	2.0
(soft)	3 oz.	2.0
Tuna	3 oz.	0.0
Turkey	3 oz.	0.0
Turkey Bacon	1 slice	0.0
Prime Rib	1 oz.	0.0

MISC.

Food	Amount	Carbohydrate Gram
Bacon Bits	1 T.	1.7
Beef Jerky	1 pce.	0.5
Buyer	1 tsp.	0.1
Cappuccino	8 oz.	24.0
Catsup	1 T.	20.0
Crouton	1 C.	22.0
Custard	1 C.	30.2
Espresso	8 oz.	0.9
Garlic	1 clove	0.9
	1 tsp.	0.6
Horseradish	1 T.	2.8
Jello (sugarfree)	1 C.	0.0
Margarine	1 tsp.	0.1
Mayo (Kraft reg.)	1 T.	0.0
Olive	1item	0.3
Olive oil	1 T.	0.0

Nuts

Food	Amount	Carbohydrate Gram
Almond	1/4 C.	8.4
Brazil (shelled/dried)	1/4 C.	4.5
Cashews (dry roasted)	1/4 C.	11.2

Food	Amount	Carbohydrate Gram
Chestnut (roasted)	1 oz.	14.0
Hazelnut	1 oz.	4.8
Macadamia (dried)	1/4 C.	4.6
Mixed	1/4 C.	5.0
Peanut (dry roasted)	1/4 C.	7.8
Peanut butter (smooth or crunchy)	1 T.	3.0
Pecan (dry roasted)	1/4 C.	6.2
Pignola	1 T	1.4
Pistachio (dry roasted)	1/4 C.	8.7
Sunflower seeds	1/4 C	7.7
Walnut (chopped black)	1/4 C	3.7

Sauces and Dips

Food	Amount	Carbohydrate Gram
Alfredo sauce	1/2 C.	10.0
Barbecue	1 T.	5.0
Bearnaise	1/2 C.	8.7
Beef gravy	1/2 C.	5.6
Cocktail	1 T.	4.5
Creamer (creamora lite liquid)	1 tsp.	20
(nondairy/FF - liquid coffee mate)	1 T.	20
(powder flavored)	1 T.	6.8
Dip (black bean)	1 T.	2.0
(Guacamole)	1 T.	1.5
(Jalapeno)	1 T.	1.5
(onion)	1 T.	20
(refried bean)	1 T.	20
Half and Half	1 T.	0.6
Hollandaise	1 T.	3.0
Hot sauce	1 tsp.	0.1
Jelly	1 T.	13.5
Maple syrup	1/2 C.	99.5
Mustard (yellow)	1 tsp.	0.5
(Grey Poupon)	1 tsp.	0.5
(Brown)	1 tsp.	0.8
Salsa	1 T.	1.0
Salad dressing (Blue cheese)	1 T.	1.1
(Caesar)	1 T.	0.5

Food	Amount	Carbohydrate Gram
(French)	1 T.	2.7
(Italian)	1 T.	1.0
(HoneyMustard)	1 T.	2.0
(Ranch)	1 T.	0.6
(Thousand ls.)	1 T.	2.3
(Vinegar&Oil)	1 T.	0.4
Spaghetti sauce	1/2 C.	19.8
Sour cream	1 T.	0.5
Soy sauce	1 T.	1.5
Sugar (granulated)	1 T.	12.5
Sweet and sour	1 T.	4.5
Tomato catsup	1 T.	2.0
(low sodium)	1 T.	4.6
(ketchup lite)	1 T.	3D
Tartar	1 T.	1.0
Tomato	1/2 C.	8.8
Whipping cream (Heavy)	1 T.	0.2
Worcestershire	1 T.	2.7

Soup

Food	Amount	Carbohydrate Gram
Chicken noodle	1 C	10.1
Chicken Broth	1 C.	.9
Chicken and Rice	1 C.	13.0
Chili beef	1 C.	30.0
Clam Chowder	1 C.	17.0
Beef stew	1 C.	15.0
Black bean	1 C.	34.0
Bouillon	1 item	1.0
Broccoli and cheese	1 C.	18.0
Corn chowder	1 C.	32.0
Cream of asparagus	1 C.	16.0
Cream of chicken	1 C.	15.0
Ham andbean	1 C.	34.0
Manhattan clam chowder	1 C.	24.0
Minestrone	1 C.	18.0
Potato	1 C.	17.0

Food	Amount	Carbohydrate Gram
Oyster stew	1 C	9.0
Split Pea	1 C.	28.0
Tomato	1 C.	12.8
Turkey Rice	1 C.	8.0
Vegetable Beef	1 C.	20.0

Spices

Food	Amount	Carbohydrate Gram
Allspice (ground)	1 tsp.	1.4
Capons	1 tsp.	0.0
Chives	1 tsp.	0.0
Coriander	1 T.	0.9
Vanilla extract	1 T.	4.3
Vinegar	1 T.	0.7

Starch

Food	Amount	Carbohydrate Gram
Bagel (plain)	1 item	38.0
(cinnamon)	1 item	39.0
Bag Chips	1 C.	44.0
Better Cheddar	6 each	4.6
Biscuit	1 item	17.0
Bread (French)	1 slice	13.0
(Italian)	1 slice	15.0
(wheat)	1 slice	11.0
(mixed grain)	1 slice	12.0
(rye)	1 slice	15.0
(sourdough)	1 slice	13.0
(white)	1 slice	33.0
(white/low calorie)	1 slice	10.0
Bread Crumbs	1/4 C.	19.5
Breadstick	1 stick	2.2
Corn tortilla	1 each	11.7
Corn chips	1 oz.	16.0
Couscous	1/2 C.	20.5
Flour tortilla	1 each	19.5
French toast	1 slice	13.0

Food	Amount	Carbohydrate Gram
Grits (yellow)	1 C.	31.5
(instant original Quaker)	1 C.	22.0
Graham cracker	3 each	15.9
Harvest Crisps oat Nabisco	6 each	9.6
Hominy	1 C.	22.0
Macaroni	1/2 C.	19.8
Melba toast	6 each	22.9
Noodles	1/2 C.	19.8
Oyster Cracker	6 item	1.8
Pancake	1 C.	82.0
Pasta	1/2 C.	19.5
Pita (white)	1 item	33.0
(wheat)	1 item	35.0
(dinner)	1 item	13.0
Popcorn	1 C.	7.9
Potato	1 item	51.0
(mashed)	1/2 C.	18.0
Potato chips	1 oz.	14.0
Pretzel	1 C.	34.0
Rice	1/2 C.	22.0
Rice Cake	1 each	7.6
Waffle	1 each	15.0
Roll (hard)	1 each	30.0
(egg)	1 each	18.2
Saltines	6 each	12.6
Stuffing	1/2 C.	14.5
Sweet potato	1 item	27.7
Wheat thins original-Nabisco	6 each	6.6

Vegetables

Food	Amount	Carbohydrate Gram
Artichoke heart	1 each	3.0
Asparagus(canned)	1 C.	6.0
(raw)	1 C.	6.0
(frzn Green Giant)	1 C.	6.0
Beets (pickled)	1 C.	37.0
(raw)	1 C	24.6
(harvard)	1 C.	44.0

Food	Amount	Carbohydrate Gram
Broccoli (frzn)	1 C.	7.8
(raw)	1 C.	4.6
Cabbage (common shredded)	1 C.	3.8
(common boiled)	1 C.	6.7
Carrot (shredded)	1/2 C.	5.1
(raw)	1 C.	21.5
(boiled)	1 C.	25.1
Cauliflower (boiled)	1 C.	5.1
Celery (raw stalk)	1 item	1.5
(diced)	1 C.	4.5
(raw)	1 C.	7.8
Collard Greens (frzn)	1 C.	4.0
(seasoned w/pork lucks)	1 C.	10.0
Corn (ear/frzn/boil)	1 item	14.1
(frzn/boil/kernel)	1/2 C.	16.5
(sweet corn canned)	1/2 C.	15.2
Cucumber (raw)	1 C.	6.5
(raw whole)	1 slice	8.3
(raw Minced)	1 C.	2.8
(pickle dill)	1 slice (2.3 oz.)	2.7
Eggplant (raw)	1 C.	4.9
(boiled)	1 C.	6.3
Mixed vegetables(frzn)	1 C.	24.0
(canned)	1 C.	15.0
(frzn Green Giant)	1 C.	15.0
Lettuce (Iceberg raw/chopped)	1 C.	1.1
(Iceberg piece)	1 piece	.5
(Romaine/raw/shredded)	1 C..	1.3
Lima Bean (raw boiled)	1 C.	127.0
Mushroom (boiled)	1 each	0.7
(raw/chopped)	1 C.	3.3
(Portabella)	1 each	1.3
Mustard Greens (frzn/boiled)	1 C.	6.0
(boiled)	1 C.	2.9
Okra (fried/batter/dip)	1 C.	11.5
(raw boiled)	1 C.	11.5
Onion (raw/chopped)	1 C.	13.8
(boiled)	1 C.	22.7

Food	Amount	Carbohydrate Gram
Parsnips	1 C.	30.5
Peppers (Green/Red/Yellow)	1 item	4.7
Radishes	1 item	0.2
Rutabagas (raw)	1 C.	101.4
(boiled drain)	1 C.	14.9
Sauerkraut (canned)	1 C.	10.1
Snap Peas (frzn)	1 C.	8.7
(raw)	1 C.	9.8
Snow Peas	1 C.	11.0
Spinach (frzn/cooked)	1 C.	10.1
(raw chopped)	1 C.	1.9
(canned)	1 C.	7.2
Squash Zucchini		
(green/zuchini/raw)	1 C.	7.0
(raw sliced)	1 C.	3.7
(frznboiled)	1 C	7.9
Acorn (raw/baked)	1 C.	29.9
Summer (raw/boiled)	1/2 C.	4.1
Winter (raw/baked)	1/2 C.	8.4
Tomato	1 item	5.7
(raw)	1 C	10.2
(juice)	1 C.	9.0
(juice low sodium)	1 C.	7.2
(paste)	1/2 C.	25.0
(paste no salt)	1/2 C.	25.0
Turnips (green)	1 C.	6.0
(boiled)	1 C.	21.0
(frzn boiled)	1 C.	8.1
(raw boiled)	1 C.	6.3
Water chestnuts (canned)	1 C.	17.0
(raw)	1 C.	29.7

RECOMMEND / AVOID LIST

Food	Recommend	Avoid
Alcohol	Dry wine Martini Liquor and soda	Mixed drinks Daiquiri Cordials Mixed drinks w/juice

** Only 2 drinks per day or less.

Mixers	Club Soda Diet Drinks (sugar-free)	Water

Food	Recommend	Avoid
*Bean	Green beans Wax bean	All beans
Beverages	Sugar free drinks Water (8 cups per day) Herbal tea Decaffeinated coffee Skim milk	Soft drinks Lemonade Juices
*Cereal	None	Cereal with cho>7 All cereal except puffed.
Cheese	All regular cheese Low fat cheese Cottage cheese (1/2 C. serve.) Low fat cottage cheese (1/2 C. serving)	No fat cheeses (if cho>2 oz.) No fat cottage cheese
Dessert	Sugar Free vanilla pudding	Chocolate, lemon & rice pudding

* Beans and Cereals may be consumed when on maintenance diet, after weight loss has been achieved. Preferably those with a low glycemic index.

Food	Recommend	Avoid
DISHES	Chicken cordon blue	Manicotti
	Chicken cacciatore	Pizza
	Fajitas (no shell)	Tamale
		Ravioli
FRUIT *	Plum, strawberries	banana, raisins
	Kiwi, cantaloupe	Grapefruit, apple
	Watermelon, tangerine	Blackberry, blueberry
	Passion fruit, peach	cherries, prunes
	Honeydew, guava	pineapple
	Raspberry, papaya, orange	

* Fruit on the maintenance diet may be eaten in recommend list and also those fruits which containing >3 grams of fiber/serving in the Avoid category

Food	Recommend	Avoid
FRUIT JUICE		
	None	All
MEAT	All meat	Meat salads prepared with sugar Ex: Chicken salad
	Tofu in limited amounts	Imitation crab meat
		Mussel
MISC.	Bacon bits, beef jerky	Cappuccino, crouton
	Espresso, garlic	Custard
	Horseradish, SF Jello	
	Olive, olive oil	
NUTS	Brazil, hazelnut	Almond, Chest nut, cashews
	Macadamia, mixed	pistachio, sunflower seeds
	Pignolia, walnut, Peanut butter	Pecan, peanuts

Food	Recommend	Avoid
SAUCES AND DIPS		
	Alfredo, Bearnaise,	Barbecue, cocktail sauce
	Half and half	Creamer
	Hollandaise, hot sauce	Jelly, maple syrup
	Salsa, blue cheese	French, honey mustard
	Caesar, mustard, sour	spaghetti sauce
	Whipping cream	Catsup, sweet and sour
	Tartar	
SOUPS	Chicken broth, bouillon	Avoid all soups unless Clear and made without rice and pasta
	Use only clear broth soup	
SPICE	All	None
STARCH	None	All
VEGETABLE		
	Asparagus,	Beets
	Broccoli, cabbage	carrot
	Cauliflower,	Corn
	Celery, collard green	mixed vegetables
	Cucumber	Lima bean
	Eggplant, lettuce	Okra, parsnips
	Mushroom, onion	vegetable juice
	Peppers, radishes,	water chestnuts
	Snow peas, spinach	
	Squash, zucchini, tomato	
	turnips	

SNACKS

Food	Serving Size	CARBOHYDRATE GRAMS
Beef Jerky	.21 oz.	1.0
Slim Jim	1 pc.	1.0
Cashews	.5 oz	4.0
Care Free Gum	1 pc.	2.0
Breath Savers	1 pc.	2.0
Cantaloupe	.5 C.	6.0
Cucumber		
w/cream cheese	1 oz.	2.0
Celery	1 stick	1.0
Broccoli	1 C.	2.0
Cauliflower	1 C.	2.0
Ranch dressing	1 T.	2.0
Sunflower seeds	1 oz.	4.0
Walnuts	1 oz.	5.0
Macadamia nuts	1 oz.	4.0
Egg	1 ea.	.6
Strawberries	.5 C.	3.0
Sweet Pepper	.5 C.	2.0
Lettuce	1 C.	.4
Radish	5 ea.	1.0
2%Cottage Cheese	.5 C.	4.0
Cream Cheese	1 oz.	1.0
FetaCheese	1 oz.	1.0

CHAPTER V.

VITAMIN AND MINERAL SUPPLEMENTS ESSENTIAL TO PROTECT YOUR ARTERIES AND BURN FAT

The recommended daily allowance of vitamins that has been formulated by The American Dietetic Association is woefully under represented. There are several important enzymatic reactions in your body that need help. Your average balanced diet, especially the one recommended by The American Dietetic Association, predominantly carbohydrates, is void of most of the important vitamins that I will speak of in this chapter.

CHROMIUM

The first important substance to help you burn fat as energy rather than store it, is Chromium. Chromium is essential in blood sugar metabolism. Chromium itself can help you lose weight and body fat even without other manipulations in your diet. A study was done with calorie diets equal in two populations of women. The only difference between the two populations was Chromium taken in doses of between 200 and 1000 mcg. in one group, and no Chromium in the other. With no difference in exercise or calorie expenditures between the two groups, the group who took the Chromium lost weight. The Chromium which was used was Chromium Picolinate. Recently, there have been advances in the bioavailability of Chromium. Chromium POLYnicotinate improved blood sugar control in diabetics, improved weight loss in obese women and improves insulin sensitivity better than Chromium Picolinate.[8]

In view of the improved bioavailability of Chromium Polynicotinate, I have recommended for my patients to prefer this type over the Chromium Picolinate. I think either will work to help improve insulin insensitivity, but there is evidence that Chromium Polynicotinate will help you lose more weight faster. The dose that has been studied has been between 200 and 1000 mcg. daily.

An investigation at the University of Texas at Austin took a group of sedentary obese women and gave them Chromium Picolinate versus Chromium POLYnicotinate. Chromium Picolinate actually showed the women increasing both fat free mass and a slight gain in fat mass.

Whereas, Chromium POLYnicotinate, also called *Nicotinate*, caused a significant reduction in body fat and lowered insulin response to oral glucose load.

Chromium is essential in patients with Type 2 diabetes and obesity. Chromium supplementation demonstrated significant benefits in glycohemoglobin, blood sugar, fasting insulin levels, and cholesterol variables. So, Chromium should be used probably by everyone for improved metabolism. I would recommend Chromium Polynicotinate between 600 mcg and 1000 mcg. daily.

ANTIOXIDANTS

The next important vitamins to take are the antioxidants. Antioxidants are vitamins that have the ability to sacrifice themselves for free radicals. Remember, that free radicals are those oxygen molecules that have lost an electron. The antioxidants will donate electrons destroying themselves in the process, but will protect your circulating LDL cholesterol from being oxidized. If the LDL cholesterol is not oxidized, it will be less likely to become atherogenic. That means it will be less likely to incorporate itself into the blood vessel wall. White blood cells will be less likely to migrate to the site of injury of a blood vessel. If you can reduce the oxidation of LDL cholesterol with a vitamin, you should do so. You can definitely reduce the oxidation of LDL cholesterol by taking the antioxidant groups which are Vitamin E, Vitamin C, Beta-carotene and Selenium. There is some recent evidence that antioxidants don't work at very high doses. In other words, you can take too much of a good thing. People taking more than 1000 I.U. of Vitamin E, may have a contradictory effect and will not get the natural antioxidant effect from Vitamin E. Vitamin C, which is really not an antioxidant, but helps replenish Vitamin E and keeps it working as an antioxidant, should be used at a dose of 500 mg. daily. Vitamin E dose should be between 200 -400 I.U. daily.

Beta-carotene and Selenium are also important antioxidants. For Beta-carotene, which is basically Vitamin A, it should be 5000 I.U. daily. Selenium, which is an important mineral to help the antioxidants work properly, should be at least 15 mcg. daily. Manganese should be used at 1.5 mg. Additional minerals that help the antioxidants function are Zinc, between 7 and 14 mg. daily, and Copper, between 1 and 2 mg. daily. This is the group of antioxidant vitamins and minerals that I think are important to replenish each day. Remember, the free radicals will not be able to destroy your arteries or cells if you have proper amounts of these vitamins.

Another important antioxidant that appears to be helpful in reducing free radical activity is Coenzyme Q10 (CoQ10). This enzyme is essential for virtually all energy production. It is a potent antioxidant and aids in maintenance of the immune system.

FOLIC ACID

Folic acid is the next important vitamin that I would take daily. Folic Acid has been found to reduce birth defects. The interesting thing is that if you start taking it after you learn you are pregnant, it is too late. The neural tube, which is the spinal cord, is formed within the first eight weeks. Neural tube defects, such as spina bifida, will already occur with increased frequency if you are not already taking Folic Acid at the time of your pregnancy. That's why it is a recommendation by the Public Health Department that all childbearing women who consider having children should take 1 mg. of folic acid daily. Remember, 1 mg. equals 1000 mcg. The reason it is important to point this out, is that over 20 years ago, Folic Acid was removed from our vitamins. The powers that be had our health in mind, but they made the wrong decision. For some time it was illegal to have folic acid in vitamins. The reason is this: Vitamin B12 and folic acid are very important to make red blood cells. Red blood cells are the essential cell in our blood that attracts and carries oxygen. If you don't have enough red blood cells, because you can't make enough red blood cells, then you are anemic.

Folic Acid and Vitamin B12 are necessary to help the cell divide. Mitosis is the biological process by which a cell doubles it's chromosomes and then splits into two, thereby dividing and making two cells from one. We multiply our red blood cells by doubling the chromosomes within the red blood cell and then the red blood cell will split into two red blood cells. Then, those red blood cells will create two more red blood cells. The vitamins that are essential to allow the red blood cells to split and divide into two red blood cells are Folic Acid and Vitamin B12.

There is a small segment of our population that loses the ability to digest and absorb Vitamin B12. Vitamin B12 has a complicated digestive process. You need a certain amount of stomach acid and a protein called intrinsic factor that is made in your stomach. It will then cart Vitamin B12 to the terminal ilium of the small intestines and Vitamin B12 will be absorbed into the blood. It will then go to the bone marrow so you can divide your red blood cells with the help of Folic Acid, and it will go to the nervous system to nourish the spinal cord. Some people who lose the ability to digest Vitamin B12 because they have disease of the terminal ilium of their small intestines or they have disease of their stomach and cannot make intrinsic factor, will become Vitamin B12 deficient. These people will eventually become anemic, and they will eventually develop forgetfulness, dementia, and problems with their balance and spinal cord. It will contribute to a process called peripheral neuropathy.

Because anemia is one of the ways the doctor can pick this up, it is important to do a hemoglobin and a hematocrit blood test, which are measurements of the red blood cell components in your blood. Folic Acid, itself, can help the red cell divide. If you didn't have Vitamin B12, but you took Folic Acid, you could continue to make your red blood cells. When your doctor heard you complaining about being forgetful and having imbalance in your feet because you had a Vitamin B12 Deficiency, and he did a blood count to see if you were anemic, he would find out that you were not anemic, if you were taking Folic Acid. Folic Acid corrects the anemia of Vitamin B12 Deficiency, but it does not correct the spinal and central nervous system abnormalities of Vitamin B12. Because of this, the powers that be, restricted Folic Acid intake in vitamins so that we would not miss Vitamin B12 deficiency. We would recognize the fact that, if you were anemic, we would test you for Vitamin B12, and then we would not miss the other conditions that Vitamin B12 causes.

This sounds great. But the problem is that Vitamin B12 Deficiency and what it causes, pernicious anemia, are rare. In my 20 years and my 100,000 patient visits, I have seen it ten times. I also consider myself smart enough to think of it if someone complains of peripheral neuropathy or dementia. But because they removed Folic Acid from the vitamins twenty years ago, there has been a climb in Neural Tube Defects and in Coronary Artery Disease. We are starting to finally realize that we need Folic Acid, and that if we miss Vitamin B12 Deficiency because of it, it is not nearly as dangerous as the birth defects and the Coronary Artery Disease that occurs WITHOUT Folic Acid.

That is why up to this point, it has been difficult to find Folic Acid at the proper dose in your vitamins. If a woman decides that she wants to have a child, she should start taking Folic Acid at 1 mg. daily right away because by the time she becomes pregnant, it is already too late to save the baby's spinal cord.

On the other hand, Folic Acid has been found to reduce homocysteine levels and thereby reduce the scarring process that occurs in a blood vessel. Homocysteine stimulates fibroblasts which stimulate collagen and scar tissue development in the blood vessel. So people who take between 1 and 5 mg. of Folic Acid appear to have reduced homocysteine levels and reduced coronary artery disease. Folic Acid is back en vogue. We'll just have to remember to check your B12 level if you get sick. But we shouldn't make you sick by withholding Folic Acid, which is what we have done over the past twenty years. Please take between 1 and 5 mg of Folic acid for your health, especially if you have coronary artery disease, want to prevent coronary artery disease or are of childbearing age.[9]

POTASSIUM

The next important mineral is Potassium. As you lose weight and lose body fat, you are going to lose water. As you lose water, you reduce your circulating potassium levels. Potassium is vital in muscle metabolism and function. You may get weak and lethargic and have pain in your muscles if you lose too much potassium from losing a lot of your body water. Please supplement your diet with at least 100 mg. of potassium daily. This can be as potassium chloride salt or potassium supplement. I wouldn't mention these ingredients in your diet if they weren't essential. I have found that through trial and error it works the best to take these right from the start.

FOR WOMEN ONLY

As an additional general recommendation for women, especially postmenopausal women, I would recommend at least 1000 to 1500 mg. of calcium daily. You cannot absorb more than 650 mg. of calcium through your intestines at one time, so this dose has to be broken up in three different settings. In other words, 500 mg., three different times during the day. I would suggest that women take Vitamin D, at lease 800 I.U. daily. Vitamin D is necessary to help the absorption of calcium through your intestines so it can be incorporated into the bone, thereby reducing your chance of Osteoporosis.

In women, estrogen replacement after menopause is also healthy. It not only improves your cholesterol parameters by increasing your HDL cholesterol, but Premarin, when taken orally, will increase tissue plasminogen activator (TPA). Remember, TPA is that circulating blood thinner that we use as the clot buster in a heart attack. It appears that Premarin takes such a long time to break down in the liver, that the liver doesn't have time to break down tissue plasminogen activator, so you have increased levels of TPA in your blood if you take Premarin. This is probably how Premarin reduces the risk of heart attack and stroke. It increases the natural clot busting or blood thinner in your blood. Interestingly enough, when you take the estrogen by patch form, it does not pass through your liver and it does not increase tissue plasminogen activator. So it may not be as effective for the prevention of coronary disease as oral preparation.[10]

FOOD SUPPLEMENTS

There are popular food supplements that can improve insulin's effect and thereby reduce insulin resistance in your body. To name a few:

(1) ALPHA - LIPOIC ACID - This is also known as ALA. This compound has been shown to significantly increase insulin stimulated uptake of glucose into cells and increase the sensitivity of insulin in patients with Adult Onset Type 2 Diabetes. The dose given was 1 gram of Alpha-Lipoic Acid dissolved in 500 milliliters of saline.

(2) OMEGA - 3 FATTY ACIDS - The most popular of these are found in fish fat, usually salmon. The most active ingredients here are eicosapentaenoic acid and docosahexenoic acid. Omega - 3 fat supplements in the dose of 35 mg. per 1 kilogram body weight have been shown to reduce blood levels of triglycerides in Type 2 Diabetics. In studies with pigs, Omega - 3 fatty acids improved insulin insensitivity.

(3) MAGNESIUM - This is an essential mineral for all our biologic processes. Over 300 enzymes are known to be activated by magnesium. Some evidence shows that 20 grams of magnesium a day in older non-insulin dependent diabetic patients improves insulin action. The problem with oral Magnesium is that it is poorly absorbed.

Of the above mentioned, the absolute essential things to take are the Antioxidant Vitamin, including Co-Enzyme Q10, because of the multiple benefits in reduction of heart disease and cancer from antioxidation. I have counted now at least 28 studies that show the benefits of antioxidants and reduction in Coronary Disease. Remember, be careful not to take too much and take it within the dosage ranges that I suggested.

The next essential vitamin is chromium. This diet probably won't work without chromium. If you are a diabetic, you should be taking chromium anyway. I think everyone should take at least 200 mcg. up to 1000 mcg. of chromium daily.

Thirdly, Potassium. Since you are going to be losing a lot of water weight, let's make sure your legs don't get weak from reducing all of your potassium through your urine.

Those three are ESSENTIAL. It is okay to add a one-a-day multiple vitamin to this, but as long as you take the three things I mentioned above, I think you will be all set to go.

ESSENTIAL VITAMIN AND MINERAL DOSES

VITAMIN E	200 - 400 I.U. daily (not above 800 I.U.)
VITAMIN C	500 - 1000 mg. daily
CHROMIUM POLYNICOTINATE	600 - 1000 mcg. daily
POTASSIUM	100 - 200 mg. daily
COENZYME Q 10	100 mg. daily

Mg. - milligrams
Mcg. - micrograms

CHAPTER VI.

CONTROVERSIES WITH THE LOW CARBOHYDRATE DIET

It is interesting to me that the more success people have losing weight and improving their blood parameters with a low carbohydrate diet, the more voluminous the attack on this diet through the news media. Dietary institutions take it upon themselves to protect us from this diet because they are concerned that we are going to ruin our heart, liver and kidneys. In the meantime, we ARE ruining our heart, liver and kidneys by being fat.

Let me take these issues and examine them for you because after this book is out, I am sure some more reports will hit the newsstands. First of all, we will examine Heart Disease. Obesity has recently been upgraded to a major risk factor for Heart Disease. Obesity was thought to be a contributing factor to developing coronary disease, but this is the first time it has been listed as a major risk factor. The other major risk factors are: cigarette smoking, hypertension, high blood cholesterol, meaning high LDL cholesterol and low HDL cholesterol, and a sedentary life-style. You should add diabetes to that list also.

The American Heart Association upgraded the status of obesity from a contributing factor to a major risk factor because scientific evidence that shows obesity's impact on heart disease risk and the increased prevalence of obesity in our population. To quote Dr. Robert H. Eckel, M.D., Vice-Chairman of the American Heart Association's Nutrition Committee and Professor of Medicine and Psychology at the Science Center in Denver, "We want to send a message to both health care providers and the public that the time has come to take obesity seriously." He continues, "Today our understanding of obesity and it's impact on Coronary Heart Disease is in it's infancy comparable to our understanding cholesterol's role in the heart in the mid 1970's. Dr. Eckel continues, "The call to action notes the increase of obesity in the American population. Obesity itself has become a lifelong disease, not a cosmetic issue or moral judgement. It is becoming a dangerous epidemic." They go on to explain at the American Heart Association conference that there are no simple answers as to why obesity is increasing at this time. Dr. Eckel was puzzled by the fact that obesity is increasing in incidence because the percentage of calories consumed as fat has been decreasing over the past decade. Their conclusion was that American's must be eating more calories overall. Their other conclusion was that Americans are more sedentary than any other population in the world.

It is interesting that when I go to Gold's Gym, I can't do my cardiovascular workout because the cardiovascular machines are very popular and always occupied. It is also interesting to me that for the most part it is fat people who are walking on the machines. I feel bad and almost want to go up to them and stop the machine and say, "Look, you're working so hard, your weight problem must be related to the type of food you are bringing in." If I didn't think I'd get arrested for stopping their cardiovascular workout, I would tell them to stop eating carbohydrates and the hard work of exercise would reap benefits. I would like to tell Dr. Eckel that it is not a surprise to me that America is getting fat despite the fact that we don't eat fat. That is exactly the problem. It is carbohydrates and it is insulin insensitivity that is ruining our health.

I have demonstrated in my own patients that if you eat more fat and protein and restrict carbohydrates, your cholesterol improves.Your HDL improves. Your total cholesterol/HDL ratio improves. No study in the world shows improvement in HDL cholesterol over 40%. The best you can do with Niacin is between 20% and 25%. Diet alone improves HDL cholesterol over 40%, close to 50%. These are improvements in HDL cholesterol that to this point in medicine, have not been achieved even with the strongest medicines to raise HDL. In fact, a low carbohydrate diet with increased fat and protein intake should be the treatment for a low HDL syndrome. I am absolutely convinced of it.

I am now getting referrals from cardiologists because they don't know what to do with the low HDL. I have seen people with cholesterols of 114 and HDL's of 20 who are having horrible coronary disease and multiple bypass surgeries. It is clear that it is not cholesterol but the TYPE of cholesterol. You need more snow plows. If this is unhealthy for your cardiovascular system, you need to explain to me why. Is there some secret potion in fat that is going to ruin someone's blood vessels? Are all the numbers that we were told to consider extremely important now irrelevant?

I think the problem is obesity and once you correct obesity, everything corrects with it and that is what this way of eating does. My job is to protect my patients. I am not going to put my patients on a diet that is going to make them worse. If this didn't work, I would know it immediately. My patients are more enthusiastic about this than I am because they have seen the improvement in their weight, their blood pressure and their cholesterol, as well as, the way they feel. Even the arthritic patients I have explained to me that their pain is gone. I didn't think I had a great explanation for this, but the more I read, the more I find that some of the inflammatory kinins that probably contribute to inflamed joints and inflamed arteries are reduced by reducing obesity.

Obesity is a major risk factor. That means it is just as important as cigarette smoking, diabetes and hypercholesterolemia as a risk factor for heart disease. In fact, I think it contributes to most of the other risk factors.

The other major change from the American Heart Association has been upgrading systolic blood pressure as a dominant cardiovascular risk factor. Remember, systolic blood pressure is the top number. The National Health and Nutrition examination survey database reveals that 25% of the U.S. population (about 43,000,000 people) have hypertension defined as a blood pressure above 140/90. In fact, at a systolic blood pressure of 140 mm of mercury, the patient's risk of developing coronary disease is nearly double that of someone with a blood pressure of 120/70. The risk was also greater in elderly people. The problem is that sometimes their vessels are so stiff that you can't get the blood pressure down without making them sick, as we discussed with Dr. William Osler's work. The major way that I know to get your blood pressure down is to reduce your obesity and to reduce your insulin resistance. Again, if you wait too long, the muscles are too stiff and musclebound in your arteries and you won't improve them. It is hard for me to fathom that losing 30 lbs. of body fat is bad for your heart. You immediately reduce a major risk factor for heart disease. You reduce insulin stimulation of the smooth muscle in your arteries so you reduce your blood pressure as much as possible , and you reverse a trend that is happening in our country towards greater obesity.

The next controversy I would like to address is kidney disease. If your kidneys are normal, protein is not going to hurt your kidneys. If your kidneys are already diseased, everything bothers your kidneys. Once the kidney disease has set in by diabetes or long-standing hypertension, the kidney, which is a filter, will probably be influenced by salt, potassium, phosphorus and protein. The key is to *prevent* the kidney disease to prevent protein leaks through the kidney. When the kidney is diseased, it leaks protein. This can start out with very small amounts called microalbuminuria. Microalbuminuria means that you are leaking small amounts of albumin through the kidney. This is due to a break in the lining of the kidney called the basement membrane. This happens probably after about five years of diabetes. Some studies claim ten years. In any event, it is important for the doctor to check urine for microalbuminuria. It is not universally accepted that if you have microalbuminuria you will advance to frank kidney failure, but the consensus is that microalbuminuria is the beginning of a progression of disease in your kidney towards kidney failure.

Why does the kidney fail in diabetes? We are not 100% sure. Probably because of the high blood sugar. Glucose or sugar and protein are very hydrophilic, the Greek word - to love water. They attract water like a magnet and iron. Wherever they go, they bring water with it. If your kidneys are filtering too much sugar because the sugar in your blood is too high, there will be an increased flow of sugar and water through your kidneys. This will also drag protein with it, so there will be an increased flow of protein. Eventually, this increased flow creates an increased pressure within the filtering tubule of the kidney called the *glomerulus*. The glomerulus will wear down and break and eventually you will have little holes in the filtering lining of the kidney and you will start leaking protein. The diseased glomeruli that are unable to filter any more will shut down and the ones that are healthy will have to increase their work of filtering this tremendous force of fluid and that will eventually knock off the rest of your filtering capabilities in the kidney. Exactly what does this in diabetes is not known. I am not quite sure why it is not known. Things are hard to prove in scientific studies, but this doesn't happen in people who have normal blood pressure and normal blood sugars. It happens 25% of the time when the blood sugar' is high, so it is logical to me that it is the high blood sugar dragging water through the kidneys in increased force.

Once you set up that situation everything can affect the filtering system of the kidney. Protein is very similar to sugar in its ability to drag water around. In fact, it is sugar and protein which has such a chemical attraction to water that along with salt, keeps the fluid in our blood vessels. Our blood vessels are porous. They are not solid tubes, so the water would leak out if you didn't have some attraction to keep it in the blood vessels. What keeps the water in our blood vessels to fill up our cardiovascular system and give us blood pressure? The answer is salt or sodium, proteins, such as albumin, made from our liver and sugar. They are all hydrophilic substances. Once your kidney is diseased, protein, sugar and phosphorus will effect the kidney function and actually increase the progression of the kidney disease. If your kidney's are normal, and you don't have these conditions, there is no way that increasing protein intake is going to ruin your kidneys.

Eating steak and eggs is not going to ruin your kidney function. You are not talking about high protein diets anyway. You are talking about NORMAL protein diets. A normal person can take between 1 and 1.3

grams of protein per kilogram per day. Someone with kidney failure should probably restrict their protein intake to between 0.6 and 0.8 grams of protein per kilogram per day. So, if you still want to lose weight and restrict your carbohydrates , you will have to count your protein grams if you have kidney failure. If you do not have kidney failure, don't worry about it. It is not going to harm your kidneys. If you have diabetes and you do not have microalbuminuria or proteinuria, which means protein in the urine, then you should prevent those conditions by getting your blood sugar down. At that point, I would not worry about protein intake. Once your kidneys are damaged, however, that process is probably irreversible for most people no matter what you do.

Normal or even slightly increased protein intake is not going to ruin a normal kidney. There is no evidence for that anywhere. If you have long-standing high blood pressure, you should have a urinalysis done by your physician. He can check for microalbuminuria with a special test of your urine. A simple dipstick of the urine will tell if you have any macroalbuminuria or high amounts of protein in your urine. Speaking of people who already have kidney disease, there is evidence that protein restriction slows the progression of chronic renal failure in experimental models. The findings from human studies are less conclusive. A number of studies in diabetic patients do, indeed, suggest that protein restriction is beneficial. These are people who already have kidney disease and protein in their urine. This however, is controversial among kidney specialists. Some kidney specialists argue that restricting protein may slow down renal disease progression, but will not stop it, so the inevitable end stage kidney failure is going to be down the road. In the process of restricting protein, you reduce your nutritional status since protein is important for your heart, your liver, your muscles, your immune system and your hormones.

It is currently controversial whether the protein restriction should be universally accepted. In 1994, came the long awaited results of the Modification of Diet in Renal Disease study which was sponsored by the National Institute of Health. In this study, non-diabetic patients with moderate renal failure or insufficiency were placed on a low protein diet with 0.6 grams per kilogram per day, and a normal protein diet which is 1.3 grams per kilogram per day. Also patients with severe kidney failure were placed on a low protein diet with 0.6 grams per kilogram per day and a very low protein diet of 0.4 grams per kilogram per day. The people with severe kidney failure were on low protein diets and lower protein diets. The people with moderate kidney failure were on low protein diets and normal protein diets. At three years of follow-up, this prospective multicenter clinical trial failed to demonstrate clearly that protein restriction benefits non-diabetic patients with moderate kidney failure of diverse etiologies. In other words, kidney failure for every other reason than diabetes was studied, and there was no clear benefit of protein restriction in those people. In patients with severe kidney failure in this study, a very low protein diet compared with a low protein diet, did not significantly slow the progression of renal disease.

The most important finding from this study was that lowering the blood pressure was the most important thing you could do for the kidney. It was much more important than protein restriction. It was most evident in African Americans who had moderate kidney failure. I think, at this point, that keeping your protein below 0.8 grams per kilogram per day if you are diabetic with kidney disease probably is the thing to do. That may change with time but for now it is the consensus. You can count your protein grams as well as your carbohydrate grams. If you don't have kidney failure or protein in the urine, don't worry about any of this. Apparently, if you have kidney failure for any other reasons, it may not help to restrict protein according to the Modification of Diet and Renal Disease study. Diabetic kidney disease may be a special case.

If I had my choice, I would get my sugar down by restricting carbohydrates because the sugar is going to ruin your heart, your blood vessels and your peripheral nerves in addition to your kidney's.

The statement by dietary institutions that a high protein diet will ruin a normal liver is unfounded. The controversy that a low carbohydrate diet will ruin your liver is really ridiculous. Your liver makes protein. It makes albumin. It makes clotting proteins. It is the source of protein production for your body. It needs protein to do this.

There are 21 amino acids which are the building blocks of protein and nine of these amino acids cannot be made by the body. They have to be supplied by your diet. They are called essential amino acids. If you don't take them in, you can't make the thousands of enzymes and proteins that go into structuring our body and making our body run. Of course, if you drink too much alcohol or have infectious diseases of the liver, which ruin the liver, then the liver can't handle protein. But taking in protein will not ruin your liver. It will make your body healthy. There is no evidence that any of these high protein intakes will cause liver failure. If your liver has already failed, just like if your kidney has already failed, then salt and protein will affect those organs because they don't function properly. If they are normal, you won't harm them by eating a low carbohydrate diet.

One of the most important investigations going on now is investigating the fat around organs. If you are fat around the middle, around your belly, then that correlates with fat around your liver, kidney and heart. You can see this in CAT scan studies. When I get a CAT scan on one of my patients who has abdominal pain and they are fat around the belly, called central obesity, you can see a lot of fat on the CAT scan and a lot of fat around and in the organs themselves. The muscle and tissue of the organs gets marbled just like a bad steak. This fat probably contributes to the disease process of those organs. If you lose central obesity you really reduce your incidence of heart disease. If your waist is thin and your fat is mostly on your hips and legs, this does not correlate with heart disease. There are no organs in your hips and legs that can be influenced by fat so that if your waist is thin, but the rest of your lower body is fat, this does not increase your risk of cardiovascular disease. It is the big belly and fat around the organs internally that increases your risk of cardiovascular disease. Many of my patients will initially lose 15 or 20 lbs. immediately after restricting carbohydrates for three months. They then notice that their weight loss hits a plateau. It really doesn't hit a plateau. The improved protein increases their muscle tone. The increased exercise improves their muscle strength but their waist size continues to shrink so they are losing their central obesity and losing their ability to create high blood pressure and heart disease.

The key is to get our waist size down. Weighing yourself is less important than the dress or belt size changes that you will see with this diet. Stop listening to the naysayers who say don't do this because it is dangerous. It is dangerous to be fat. You can stop being fat if you restrict carbohydrates.

CHAPTER VII

EXERCISE FOR FAT LOSS AND GOOD HEALTH

There is no getting around it, you need to exercise for a healthy trim body. In my practice of medicine, I've heard every excuse imaginable. The excuses do not matter! YOU MUST EXERCISE. Your muscles and bones thrive on exercise and will wither away without it. The frustrating thing is getting started when you feel hopelessly out of shape and weak. Let me help you. First of all, you will lose fat with this insulin regulating diet whether or not you exercise. You will not however reap the maximum benefits of this diet *unless* you exercise.

The first thing that I would suggest you do is walking. Studies show improved cardiac function, reduced cardiac failure and longevity with walking. The important thing to remember is that you need to walk ONE HOUR a day for at least 6 days a week. Walking twenty minutes will not accomplish our goal of improved cardiovascular fitness. If you do not want to spend an hour walking for your hearts sake, then jogging for 30 minutes will do it. If you jog for 30 minutes FOUR times a week, you will equal the cardiovascular or aerobic effect of walking for one hour SIX days a week. Anything less and you will not get cardiovascular and fat losing benefits.

REMEMBER, please, if you plan on jogging and you are over 50 years old, you must have an EXERCISE STRESS TEST. This is essential to determine if there is any underlying silent coronary artery disease. If you do not do a stress test, you will not find silent blockages in your arteries. Believe me, they are very quiet and asymptomatic until they jump up and bite you with a sudden death or heart attack. Sixty percent of people who die of a heart attack, die before they can get to a hospital. With balloon angioplasty, coronary stent placement and bypass surgery, we can fix anything. But, we cannot fix a dead person. So, please, have a stress test. I have uncovered hundreds of asymptomatic blocked arteries this year alone with stress tests. Patients often ask me if it is safe to have a stress test. It is safer to exercise with a doctor watching you while you are hooked up to a cardiac monitor, than to carry groceries upstairs with severely blocked arteries and with no clue that they are blocked.

Anaerobic exercise or resistance training is also vital to a healthy body.

Building strength and muscle through weight lifting and Cybex-type machines will tone your body and improve your strength. Your energy will soar if you combined weight training with walking or endurance training. Endurance training increases cardiovascular fitness. Resistance or weight training will decrease circulating insulin levels, increase growth hormone levels and glucogen levels. Combine these two methods of exercise and your body will feel brand new.

I suggest joining a gym and getting a personal trainer for a session or two if you do not know how to weight train. Please do not be intimidated by the gym. It is critical for you to get into a regular routine of exercise. The magazine Muscle & Fitness by Joe Weider, is an excellent source of information on the how and why of weight training.

Cross Training is a term used for those who combine endurance exercise (walking, jogging, stationery bike) with resistance training. This combination of training methods was studied recently and found to reduce the markers of insulin resistance. Remember the markers of insulin resistance (high blood pressure, intra abdominal body fat, high LDL cholesterol, low HDL cholesterol and hyperinsulinism)can kill you.

The study examined the effects of combined resistance training (8 exercises, 4 sets of each exercise, 8 - 12 repetitions in a set) in a single session. They did this three times per week. The endurance training was an exercise bike or walking for 30 minutes at 60 - 70% of maximum predicted heart rate. Maximum predicted heart rate is is the number 220 minus your age. (220-40 = 180). For a 40 year old, his or her maximum predicted heart rate is 180. This combined cross training was compared to endurance training alone. Endurance training improved all the markers of insulin resistance and body composition. Strength training is additive to endurance training in its benefits for change in percent fat, insulin concentration in blood, systolic blood pressure, triglycerides and blood sugar .[11]

If you combined these training recommendations with the Hickey recommended diet, you can't help but transform your body. But you have to get started. Do not be discouraged by your current shape.

When I was studying Karate at age 36 and became discouraged because I cound not kick my leg up as high as the younger students, my Sensei (teacher) gave me some great advice. He explained; Zen proverb teaches that it is not the PRODUCT but the PROCESS. If you concentrate on the PRODUCT (height of kick, weight loss, muscle gain, whatever) you will set early deadlines and discouraging goals. Concentrate on the PROCESS and you will succeed.

Just get the process started. Give the new way of eating and exercise a chance, and you will be happier and healthier.

DR . HICKEY'S EXERCISE PRESCRIPTION

BASED ON

EXERCISE PHYSIOLOGY STUDIES

AEROBIC ENDURANCE TRAINING

Walk one hour a day ..... 6 days a week

or

Jogging 30 minutes a day ..... 4 days a week

Stationary Bike for one hour, 6 days a week is not as good as walking, but is a close second.

ANAEROBIC STRENGTH TRAINING

Weight lifting or exercise machines of all the major muscle groups: Chest, Shoulders, Back, Buttocks, Legs and Abdomen, three times a week. The frequency of THREE TIMES A WEEK is important. Exercised muscle starts the shrinking or atrophy process 72 hours after exercise. Imagine how atrophied your muscles are, if you have never exercised? The good news, if stimulated properly, they will begin to grow even up to the age of 75 years.

If you exercise the muscles every 72 hours, they will not begin the shrinking or atrophy process. You cannot expect your muscles and bones to carry you around and function efficiently if you do not nourish them. Nothing nourishes muscles better than weight training and protein intake.

CHAPTER VIII.

REFERENCES

A. THE GLYCEMIC INDEX OF FOODS

This measures how high and how fast the blood sugar (glucose) rises after eating these foods. The standard (glycemic index of 100%) was set by Dr. Jenkins et al who tested foods against pure sugar (glucose) ingestion.

RAPID INDUCERS OF INSULIN

GLYCEMIC INDEX GREATER OR EQUAL TO 100%

Corn Flakes
Rice Krispies
Puffed Wheat
Weetabix
Instant White Rice
Millet
Tofu Ice Cream
White Bread
40 % Bran Flakes
Puffed Rice
Maltose (Beer)
French Bread
Instant Potato
Puffed Rice Cakes
Glucose
Whole Wheat Bread

GLYCEMIC INDEX BETWEEN 90% AND 99%

Grape-nuts
Carrots
Barley
Muesli
Parsnips
Shredded Wheat
Corn Chips
Apricots

GLYCEMIC INDEX BETWEEN 80% AND 89%

White Rice
Brown Rice
White Potato
Corn
Rye (whole-meal)
Shortbread
Rolled Oats
Oat Bran

Rye Crisps
Honey

Fruits:
Banana
Papaya
Mango
Raisins

GLYCEMIC INDEX BETWEEN 70% AND 79%

Kidney Beans
All-bran
Oatmeal Cookies

MODERATE INDUCERS OF INSULIN

GLYCEMIC INDEX BETWEEN 60% AND 69%

Pasta (white and whole-wheat)
Pinto Beans
Apple Juice
Beets

Rye (pumpernickel)
Wheat Kernels
Apple Sauce

GLYCEMIC INDEX BETWEEN 50% AND 59%

Peas
Table sugar (sucrose)
Yams
Custard
Dried White Beans

Oranges
Orange juice
Baked beans
Navy beans
Potato Chips

GLYCEMIC INDEX BETWEEN 40% AND 49%

Lima Beans
Sponge Cake
Sweet potato

Oatmeal (slow cooking kind)
Butter beans
Grapes

REDUCED INSULIN SECRETION

Stay under this level for snacks

GLYCEMIC INDEX BETWEEN 30% AND 39%

Apples
Pears
Peaches
Whole grain rye bread
Lentils
Black-eyed Peas
Tomato Soup
Ice Cream with fat
Milk -Skim
Milk -Whole
Yogurt

GLYCEMIC INDEX BETWEEN 20% AND 29%

Cherries
Plums
Grapefruit
Fructose

GLYCEMIC INDEX BETWEEN 10% AND 19%

Soybeans
Peanuts*

* Peanuts have high fat content that slows down the carbohydrate sugar absorption into the blood.

FOODS THAT WILL NOT RAISE BLOOD SUGAR SIGNIFICANTLY

Broccoli
Brussels Sprouts
Green Peppers
Onions
Eggs
Cheese
Half and Half
Whipped Cream
Meat (beef)
Chicken
Fish
Turkey
Shellfish
Pork grinds (skins)
Salad greens
Oil and Vinegar

BODY MASS INDEX DETERMINATION

How do you determine if you are:

1. Overweight

2. Obese

3. Morbidly Obese

The new Federal Guidelines define this in terms of your BODY MASS INDEX.

BODY MASS INDEX of 25 or HIGHER is OVERWEIGHT.
BODY MASS INDEX of 30 or HIGHER is OBESE.
BODY MASS INDEX of 40 or HIGHER is MORBIDLY OBESE.

CALCULATION OF BODY MASS INDEX

$$\text{BODY MASS INDEX} = \frac{\text{Body weight in kilograms}}{\text{Height in meters squared}}$$

One kilogram = 2.2 lbs
One Meter = 39 inches
Squared means the product of a quantity multiplied by itself

EXAMPLE (Get your calculator ready)

A person is 6 feet 2 inches, 220 lbs.

Height: 6 x 12 = 72 inches in 6 feet
+ 2 inches = 74 inches

Divide 74 inches by 39 inches/meter and you get 1.89 meters.

The height in meters is 1.89

Square this by multiplying it by itself:

1.89 x 1.89 = 3.58 meters squared.

That persons height in meters is 74 inches ÷ 39 = 1.89 meters
Height in meters squared is 1.89 x 1.89 = 3.58 meters squared.

BODY WEIGHT IN KILOGRAMS

2.2 lbs = 1 kilogram
220 lbs / 2.2 = 100 kilograms

BODY MASS FOR THAT PERSON IS:

$$\frac{\text{100 Kilograms}}{\text{3.58 meters squared}} = 27.9$$

BMI = 27.9

This person is classified as overweight, but not obese (BMI of 30 or greater)

The evidence is clear that the risk of cardiovascular disease and other diseases starts to rise at a BMI of 25 or higher. The risk of death increases as the BMI reaches or surpasses 30. Normal BMI is between 18.5 and 24.9.

WAIST MEASUREMENTS

People who are very muscular may have high BMI'S. Waist measurements can help to separate the obese.

Waist measurement is taken at the navel (umbilicus). Take this measurement on bare skin. Do not let the tape measure pinch the skin, but get the tape snug.

The new guidelines say that people with BMI 's of 25 to 35, men with waist measurements of 40 inches or more, and women with waist measurements of 35 inches or more, face an increase in health problems.

EPILOGUE

GET THE PROCESS STARTED

I have tried to put in this book all of my experiences in the battle against heart disease, obesity, hypertension and diabetes. This philosophy and study has been the result of accumulation of experiences and failures over many years. But the struggle to find answers has borne fruit.

I take my Gift of Healing from God, my father, very seriously. I have prayed that He would guide me in my advice to you.

I wish you all the best in your pursuit of good health!

God Bless You,

Joseph T. Hickey, M.D.

FOOTNOTES

1. Badimon, J.J. et al - High Density Lipoprotein Plasma Fractions Inhibit Aortic Fatty Streaks in Cholesterol Fed Rabbits. LAB INVEST 60:455, 1989

2. Badimon, J.J. et al - J: INVEST 85: 12/34 90

3. Knopp, R.H. et al - JAMA 1997; 278: 1509 - 1515

4. Alderman, M.H. et al - Lancet 351: 781 - 785, 1998.

5. Stampfer, M.J., et al - A Perspective Study of Cholesterol APO Lipoproteins, and the Risk of Myocardial infarction. The New England Journal of Medicine 3/25: 373, 1991

6. Ridker, P.M. et al - C-reactive Protein Adds to the Predictive Valve of Total and HDL Cholesterol in Determining Risk of First Myocardial Infarction. Circulation May 26, 1998; 97: 2007 - 11.

7. Gurfinkel, E., et al. Lancet 1997; 350: 404-.. 407

8. Grant, K.E, et al - Chromium and Exercise Training Effect on Obese Women. Medicine and Science in Sports and Exercise 29: 992 - 998, 1997

9. Malinow, M.R. et al - Reduction of Plasma Homocystine Levels by breakfast cereal fortified with folic acid in patients with Coronary Artery Disease, New England Journal of Medicine, 4/9/98, Volume 338, #15

10. Hormone therapy and fibrinolysis KoK, FL, New England Journal of Medicine, 1997, 336683 - 90.

11. Wallace, M.D., et al - Medicine and Science in Sports and Exercise, 20:1170-1175, 1997